KT-419-995

The
Insomniac's
Best Friend

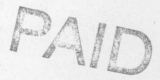

Also by Lynda Brown:

Fresh Thoughts on Food (Chatto & Windus)
The Cook's Garden (Century)
BBC Vegetables for Small Gardens (BBC Books)
The Modern Cook's Manual (Michael Joseph; Penguin)
The Shopper's Guide to Organic Food (Fourth Estate)
Organic Living (Dorling Kindersley)
The New Shopper's Guide to Organic Food (Fourth Estate)

The
Insomniac's
Best Friend

**How to get a better
night's sleep**

LYNDA BROWN

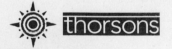

thorsons

Thorsons
An Imprint of HarperCollins*Publishers*
77–85 Fulham Palace Road,
Hammersmith,
London W6 8JB

The website address is: www.thorsonselement.com

-☼- thorsons ™

and *Thorsons* are trademarks of
HarperCollins*Publishers* Ltd

Published by Thorsons 2004

10 9 8 7 6 5 4 3 2 1

Cartoons by Harry Venning

A catalogue record for this book is
available from the British Library

ISBN 0 00 716385 1

Printed and bound in Great Britain by
Creative Print and Design (Wales), Ebbw Vale

For Christiane, with love

Contents

PART 4
Sleeping directory and resources

Preface

How it all started ...

If I look back, I guess my insomnia had been coming on for years. Not sleeping well had become part of my daily life – due, I reasoned, to the fact that, like most people today, I push myself hard. It got gradually worse. Writing two books back to back didn't help – stress levels went sky-high. But I didn't bargain for the aftermath. I took time off – and insomnia hit hard. My sleep got so bad that I began to have nights with no sleep. As insomniacs know only too well, being dog-tired yet not being able to sleep seriously does your head in – not to mention your life. Up until this time I had not used the word 'insomniac'. Like countless thousands of people who suffer severe sleep deprivation, you say to yourself 'It'll all be better tomorrow.' There is also an inexplicable shame with admitting you can't sleep. It sort of says you've failed in some way. And anyway, although we're all familiar with the word, how do we know whether clinically we are an insomniac or not? A quick search on the internet soon solved that: by any definition, I was a chronic insomniac.

Admitting I had insomnia to myself – and gradually to the rest of the world – was the first empowering step I took. Sure, people change their attitude to you (rather like depression, insomnia belongs to that underworld of darkness which makes everyone else feel uncomfortable, for a variety of reasons), but it also puts you in charge of doing something about it, more than dabbing lavender on your pillow, breathing deeply, having hot baths and all the rest of the necessary rituals you collect along the way.

I started to buy books on insomnia, dabbled in anti-depressants and for six months existed on sleeping pills. I went into obsessional over-drive about it, what it was doing to my health, and how was I ever going to claw myself out of the pit? I shovelled anxiety on myself like it was going out of style. I landed up with depression and for a time lived the life of a mole; I still, largely, live the life of a monk.

Without doubt, coping with insomnia has been the trial of my life (quite literally, as it happens). But the biggest (and nicest) surprise was to discover I was part of an unofficial club – admit you're an insomniac or can't sleep, and all of a sudden people you never dreamed had problems with being able to sleep come out as well. I also discovered that talking to fellow insomniacs was wonderfully liberating and utterly comforting: find yourself a fellow sleep-deprived soul and immediately you don't seem so alone and helpless.

Gradually things got a little better (an insomniac, like an alcoholic, takes things one day at a time; and where sleep is concerned, we always hedge our bets). By lowering my expectations of how much sleep I needed, I managed to control most of the self-induced anxieties which had helped it spiral in the first place. I weaned myself off sleeping pills, tackled stress head-on as best I could, went to see a sleep specialist, and tried various complementary therapies. I also had to truly acknowledge that chronic insomnia is a mind–body phenomenon, and that my insomnia at least was (and is) a wake-up call. That meant having to address a fair number of life issues. The result is that most of the time I can, and do, function as a human being once more – the first step back to normality we should all be able to achieve.

Though I cannot yet call myself a 'normal' sleeper (I average around 4–5 hours, and still wake up more than I would wish for), I generally do sleep better – my sleep disturbs me less and is far less disturbed. I do get blips, but these days try not to worry about them. I am also a different person, someone who understands herself, I hope, a little bit better. I am learning, too, to appreciate the little things more, and worry about what can seem like the big things less.

So, what began as a determination to get more sleep, for me has ended up as much a journey of self-exploration. Along the way I have also learned an awful lot about sleep and not sleeping, and now view it as one of the most important health and well-being issues of our day; how we should each take the responsibility for our own sleep seriously; and how, ultimately, we can only do it for ourselves.

I have also discovered that, though there is no single cure, there *is* an answer for everyone, and that no one *needs* to suffer from sleep deprivation. There *is* lots of tlc, comfort, support, solidarity, strategies for dealing with lack of sleep and good advice out there. Physicians have discovered as well that patients who are given information so that they can make sense of their problem, shed a lot of the fear and anxiety surrounding it. This is a hugely positive help in its own right, and is basically what this book is about and why I wrote it. My sincerest hope is that it will help and be of benefit to you.

Sweet dreams!

z z z z

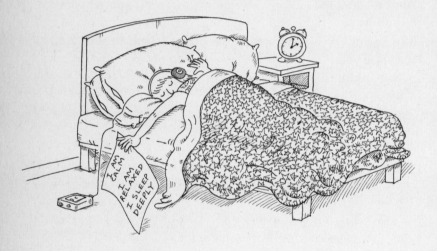

Introduction

Welcome to the club

> Without Thee what is all the morning' wealth?
> Come, blessed barrier between day and day,
> Dear mother of fresh thoughts and joyous health!
> **William Wordsworth,** *To sleep*

Do you worry about your sleep? Does not sleeping well affect your waking day? Your job? Your relationships? Does it get you down and make you anxious or depressed? Or are you just plain dog-tired? … Do you long for more sleep? Are you obsessive about getting more of it? Do you just put up with it? Or would you like to try and do something about it? Do Wordsworth's words strike a chord for you? If the answer is yes to some or all of these questions, then this book has been written for you.

There are thousands, if not millions, of people for whom sleep is a nightly struggle either some or most of the time. Even if we sleep well, almost everyone will experience the nightmare of sleepless nights, tossing and turning for no apparent reason. Many people, too, are forced into disruptive sleep due to their job or circumstances – think of shift-workers, lorry drivers, those in the health profession, pilots and cabin crews, new mums and carers, all of whom have to accept or resign themselves to sleep-deprivation as part of life.

Sometimes we can't help not sleeping well: as we know, almost any human activity involving stress, and many that don't (winning the pools or falling in love, for example) can play havoc with our sleep. Electricity did away with the natural distinction between day

z z z z

and night, and hence our natural sleep pattern which, roughly speaking, is to be awake when it's light and asleep when it's dark. But that is nothing compared to the 24-hour, go-anywhere-do-anything-anytime world we live in now, where jet-lag and all-night movies (and pizzas) are part of everyday life.

So, sleepwise, the cards are stacked against us. That wouldn't be a problem if over and above the biological necessity to sleep, lack of it makes you feel literally so deprived. Sleep is nature's built-in happy pill. And just as good sleep is our natural birthright – we are all born with an innate ability to sleep as we wish – there's a kind of natural injustice if we don't sleep well. Not to mention the frustration and generally miserable side-effects that lack of sleep, and in particular insomnia, induces.

But that is just the beginning. Probably the most frustrating thing about sleep is its utterly elusive nature. You can't see it, touch it, feel it, and because it's an unconscious activity, though scientists can measure the brain's sleep waves, which tell you something about its physiology, because we can't access it with our waking conscious brain, we can't begin to make sense of it. Which maybe is why, though mankind has been pondering about its nature since the Ancient Greeks, the science of sleep is still in its infancy and sleep scientists cheerfully admit they still don't understand that much about it. Worse still is the lack of recognition by either governments or the medical profession generally that good sleep is vital for the health of a nation, and that bad sleep is costing us all a fortune. If as much money was devoted to educating the public about the benefits of good sleep and how to sleep well, and helping those of us who suffer acutely from sleep problems, as there is on, say, preventing heart disease, we would all probably be happier, healthier, more productive and more successful.

As things stand, we must struggle on as best we can. Which is where I sincerely hope this book will help. It's first and foremost a grassroots book, based on a belief that just as we have become streetwise, we need to become 'sleepwise' from, as it were, the ground up. And to do that we need to help each other to help ourselves. Being an insomniac is a heavy, lonely burden, but sharing it with others, and learning from each other's experiences, lightens the load and opens new doors to overcoming it. So for all of you who don't just worry, but *care* about your sleep, welcome to the club – together we can crack it.

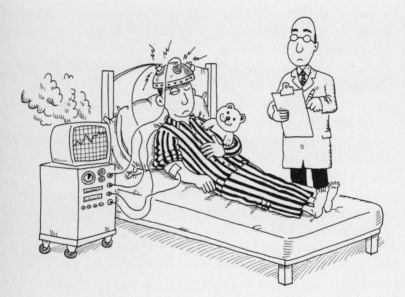

PART 1

What's all the fuss about?

Before we begin ...

This section deals with the nuts and bolts of sleep as currently understood. You may well come to the conclusion that it expresses or explains all you need to know about sleep. Which is precisely what *I* thought, too. It isn't. Sleep is a mirror to your waking life. How you sleep or don't sleep is shaped by who you are, your upbringing and childhood, and your 'journey' through life. So don't reach any final conclusions yet, at least until you've read Part 2 and the other interpretations and explanations peppered throughout this book that will help you to see that we each play centre-stage in the great drama called sleep.

z z z z

Sleep

Balm of hurt minds, great nature's second course,
Chief nourisher in life's feast.
Shakespeare, *Macbeth*, Act II

We spend a third of our lives asleep. It is one of the most important, intimate and pleasurable activities we engage in, yet two things rapidly become clear: Nobody really understands what sleep is or why we need it. It remains one of life's great mysteries.

Scientists now broadly know what happens to brain waves when we sleep, we know that sleep is necessary for survival, we know it rests, energizes and revives us, makes us feel good, alert and able to cope with our waking lives – but scientists are far from having the complete picture. Understandably, it's not been a popular study for scientific research (would you willingly deprive yourself of sleep to study others thrashing around in the middle of the night desperately trying to get some?). Nor has it been acknowledged enough among medical circles. Sleep research, for example, is desperately under-funded. As a result, the science of sleep is still very new. That we have sleep laboratories at all is thanks in part to two pioneering American sleep scientists and founding fathers of modern sleep research in the 1950s and 1960s: Nathaniel Kleitman and William C. Dement.

The only thing we do know for certain is that sleep is highly complex and involves a multitude of physiological and chemical changes. The natural mechanisms of sleep, for example, are governed by such things as body temperature, circadian rhythms, hormonal release, and genetic background – and that's before you even start on how what's happening in your life (or bedroom) and your medical history impinge on your sleep.

z z z z

From a waking person's viewpoint, however, it's idiotically simple: sleep is simply not being awake. Dreams apart, what you most experience is the non-experience of oblivion. Frankly, if you are sleep-deprived or an insomniac, this is all you really care about and desire.

The point about understanding the rudiments of sleep, however, is that it's the first step to empowerment. In other words, understand the beast and you can begin to control it. It will also help you sleep better – sleep scientists have done studies to prove it: if you need any more encouragement, one sleep study found that increasing patients' knowledge of sleep patterns reduced their wakefulness by 50 per cent.

What happens when we sleep?

Lots, in fact. Sleep is a dynamic state which has a life of its own. Though physically we seem to be, and are, at rest (except for occasional twitching and eye movements), your brain views sleep very differently. Your brain literally buzzes during sleep, and though your body clock, for example, largely determines what kind of sleeper you are, it's what happens to your brain waves that determines the quality of your sleep – and with sleep, as with most things in life, it's quality rather than quantity that counts.

During sleep your brain produces a series of distinct brain waves, shown in the graph opposite. These determine what kind of sleep you are actually experiencing. They repeat themselves to form sleep cycles, each lasting around 60 minutes in babies and 90 minutes in adults, called the *ultradian rhythm*. During a night a normal sleeper can expect to go through 4–5 cycles. In turn, each sleep cycle goes through 5 distinct phases, referred to as the stages of sleep.

The graph shows the average duration of each stage. The EEG recordings to the right of the graph depict brain activity and also eye and muscle activity.

Stages of Sleep

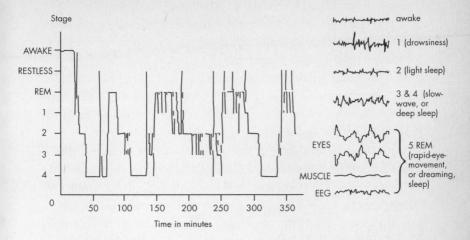

Source: *Beating Insomnia*

For practical purposes, there are two sorts of sleep. The first four stages of sleep are known as non-REM sleep (NREM). The generally accepted view is that the body repairs and regenerates itself during this sleep. In contrast, stage 5, REM (Rapid Eye Movement) sleep, also known as dreaming sleep, is thought to be where learning is processed (which is why babies spend so much time in REM sleep) as the brain sorts out its day, downloading life, filing it away and putting it back together again. It acts as a kind of safety-valve for your consciousness, and is as different to non-REM sleep as chalk is to cheese. To put it crudely, non-REM sleep fixes your body, REM sleep fixes your mind and brain. At least that's the accepted view. Recent research is beginning to re-evaluate REM sleep, in particular whether we do actually need it for our mental health. Which is comforting to know. Similar questions are being asked about NREM sleep. For example, repair and restoration of the body organs is equally effective during relaxed wakefulness. This doesn't bring us closer to the real meaning or function of sleep, but is another soothing thought for those of us living without our daily quota.

During the early parts of the night you spend more time in NREM and less time in REM sleep. There is an ongoing debate about how much core sleep we need, whether stage 1 and 2 are really vital, or just fillers, and whether REM sleep is optional.

If you don't get enough core sleep (the really deep, stage 3 and 4 stuff), for example, the brain will do its utmost to make it up, but will only make up half of any lost REM sleep. As the night progresses, sleep is lighter, you wake up more and spend more time in REM sleep. By early morning almost all your sleep is REM sleep – which is why you can often remember your dreams at this time rather than in the middle of the night.

If this sounds complicated, think of sleep as a CD with 5 tracks. The first two are Beethoven's *Moonlight Sonata* (or substitute your favourite piece of fulsomely tranquil music), the second two Gregorian chants, and the fifth a rap – and you've got it. In reality, you dip in and out of the five stages. The time each person spends in each stage varies, but generally speaking, a normal sleeping night shakes down like this:

Drowsiness

You begin your journey into sleep by first experiencing drowsiness. This is the feeling of being pleasantly sleepy. You close your eyes, your mind begins to wander and your body relaxes. Your brain waves begin to change from the rapid beta waves (15–25 Hz) of wakefulness to slower, sleepier alpha waves (8–11 Hz). Alpha waves also characterize relaxed wakefulness. Normal sleepers will spend up to 15 minutes or so being nicely drowsy before they fall asleep.

Stage 1: Light sleep

This is that hazy, lazy, crazy halfway world between sleep and being awake. Your body relaxes even more, respiration, heart rate and body temperature drop, and your thoughts become more fragmented. Alpha waves, meanwhile, give way to even slower theta waves (4–7 Hz). If you see someone 'nodding off', this is stage 1. As we know if someone wakes us up, or we wake someone else up in this stage, we wake up easily, experience momentarily disorientation and usually deny (sometimes hotly) having been asleep at all. This stage

z z z z

usually lasts a few minutes and accounts for around 5 per cent of sleep time.

Stage 2: True sleep

This is the first stage of the sleep you know nothing about, and accounts for the largest slice (around 45 per cent) of human sleep. During this time your brain begins to emit a regular jagged pattern known as sleep spindles and K complexes, unique to sleep – and interpreted by sleep scientists as the brain's attempt to retain some semblance of awareness before you reach the next stage, deep sleep. For this reason, stage 2 sleep is still regarded as light sleep – in other words, it doesn't take much to wake you up, but when you do so you are likely to feel groggy. Unless, of course, you're an insomniac, when you will probably feel bright as a button while you groan inwardly. This phase usually lasts 30–45 minutes, but can be much shorter.

The first two stages of sleep, collectively known as 'light sleep', account for about 50 per cent of total sleep time

Stages 3 and 4: Deep sleep

The holy grail of sleep. You are now profoundly asleep, or out for the count, as we would say. During stage 3, which accounts for around 7 per cent of total sleep, theta waves, sleep spindles and K complexes are still present, but give way to the slowest brain waves of all, delta waves (less than 3.5 Hz). Stage 3 sleep is typically made up of around 50 per cent theta waves. More than this and you have crossed over the threshold and entered stage 4 sleep. You are now deeply asleep – only an earthquake will wake you. Physiologically, you are literally just ticking over as oxygen consumption, heart rate, breathing and so on reach their lowest levels and your muscles become virtually comatose. It is now that the all-important growth hormone is released, necessary for cell regeneration, building new tissue and repairing damaged ones. Children and adolescents may spend up to 45 minutes in deep sleep, adults much less. Then sleep spindles and

K complexes re-emerge, and we revert to a few minutes of stage 3 sleep, before we begin the final phase of the cycle, REM sleep.

Deep sleep accounts for about 25 per cent total sleep time

Stage 5: REM (Rapid Eye Movement) sleep

Or where the fun starts. REM sleep is dream sleep or, more accurately, when we have our most vivid dreams. Though you are not conscious, brain and body are all of a sudden very active. Your eyes dart about – hence its name – while your heart rate, breathing rate and blood pressure all rise, and can be erratic (how often have you woken from a disturbing dream to find your heart thumping?). Brain waves change dramatically, becoming a heady mixture of theta, alpha and beta waves. Apart from finger and facial twitching, your muscles become paralysed, thus neatly preventing you from acting out your dreams. The well-known exception to this general state is the penis, which is why men frequently experience erections in the night (sorry, girls, it has nothing to do with you). The clitoris can also become engorged – which is why, I presume, we can also get the hots and experience orgasms in our sleep, too. REM sleep is an adventure. No wonder we wake easily from this sleep.

REM sleep also accounts for around 25 per cent of total sleep time

Stage 1 and stage 3 are transition phases, acting as doorways to true sleep and deep sleep. If you miss out on sleep, it's the lighter stages of sleep (1 and 2) that tend to be lost. The body will always do its best to catch up on deep sleep first, then REM sleep.

One final sleep-worthy point. Though this scientific classification of sleep into 5 stages is what you will read in every book on sleep, it's worth pointing out that though it has been used for over 40 years, and has enabled sleep laboratories to compare their results world-wide, sleep scientists agree that in real life even normal sleepers don't adhere to the theoretical model perfectly. In short, if you feel your sleep pattern is not doing what it's supposed to, don't worry too much. You are not alone.

z z z z

How much sleep do we need?

If you're an insomniac or not sleeping, one of the best and most comforting things to know is there seems little consensus about how much sleep we as human beings actually need. The second most comforting thing to know is that one thing scientists do agree on is that everyone's requirements for sleep are different. Advanced meditators and yogis, for example, sleep far less than other people, but do not suffer sleep deprivation. Indeed, they can achieve the same replenishment and mental and physical restoration through meditation and deep relaxation as most of us experience only by getting regular deep sleep.

The amount of sleep we need also changes through life (see below) and how much sleep you do or don't get can be conditioned by inducing good sleep habits from birth (new mums take note). Like everything else in life, too, sleep is in effect as much a lifestyle phenomena as a biological necessity, and what we view as 'normal' has been conditioned as much by culture and technology.

One thing is certain: the myth of eight hours sleep is just that. Generally speaking, adult human beings seem to like getting between 6 and 9 hours' sleep. If there is a norm, it seems to average out at $6^{1}/2$ hours. So-called 'short sleepers' require far less sleep than most of us (fewer than 6 hours), and so-called 'long sleepers' require more (9 hours or more), though this is rare. Whether you're an insomniac or not, the simplest way to determine how much sleep you need is not to measure the hours but to follow Professor Chris Idzikowski's advice: *Listen to your body.*

Generally speaking, if you fall asleep quickly, your sleep is pretty well unbroken and you get up feeling refreshed, bright and alert, your sleep is fine. If you regularly get 6 to 7 hours' sleep you can also be comforted by the findings of a 6-year Californian study involving 1 million people, which showed that people who slept for 6 to 7 hours lived longer than people who slept for 8 hours or more. I should point out that this study has caused much controversy, but does wonders for morale.

z Z z z

Sleep through the ages

Sleep patterns change throughout our lives. There are many exceptions (and we will all know some) but generally speaking:

Newborn babies	16–18 hours per day
Young children (aged 3–4)	12 hours
Older children (5–12)	10 hours
Teenagers	8 hours
Adults	7 hours

As we get older we tend to sleep less – dropping to around 6½ hours by the time we're in our seventies. As one doctor comments, it's pointless fighting this. If you find yourself progressively waking up earlier as you get older, his advice is to get up and do something constructive.

The quality of your sleep also varies with age:

Babies and young children

Babies spend half their sleep in REM sleep, compared to the 25 per cent of the time adults spend in REM sleep. Though I know parents who wouldn't agree, childhood sleep is often referred to as the golden age of sleep, where sleep problems are, generally speaking, non-existent. Because this is the age when we grow most rapidly, young children's sleep is mainly deep sleep.

Teenagers

Teens need as much sleep as children, but the sheer force of hormonal changes released at this time can play havoc with sleep patterns. If you have teenage children, let them sleep: physical growth and development need good sleep, whilst sleep debt can impair their learning ability.

Middle-age and beyond

Middle-age is crunch time. This is when we routinely get less deep sleep, sleep more lightly, and wake up more frequently and for longer intervals. Middle-aged insomniacs take comfort. As many

z z z z

elderly people know only too well, by the time we reach our seventies we enjoy virtually no deep sleep and an awful lot of napping. And you can blame this, apparently – all other things being equal – on changing circadian rhythms.

Good sleep and bad sleep

Good sleep is unbroken sleep. It is the ability to be able to fall asleep easily when you are tired, to have undisturbed sleep, and to wake when you need to – i.e., when your body and brain have had enough sleep, so that you wake up refreshed.

Bad sleep is the opposite, and is what insomniacs and poor sleepers are lumbered with. Good sleep brings consummate joy; bad sleep is a consummate pain.

Naps

If sleep scientists had their way, we would all learn the ability to nap, enlightened employers would provide napping rooms (many an insomniac has had to resort to the toilet as a refuge to help get them through the working day), and to be 'caught napping' would be encouraged rather than frowned upon and taken as a sign of weakness or laziness. Famous nappers such as President Bush and Winston Churchill have helped make 'power napping' respectable, but there's a long way to go before napping gets the credit it deserves.

In our 24-hour society, napping could be the life-line we all need. For insomniacs, napping is the fastest way to recover some of your sleep debt. Sleep guru William C Dement, a napping crusader, describes it as the most important and effective tool for dealing with sleep crises, and is convinced that naps can make you smarter, faster and safer than you would be without them. Grab any opportunity you can. They do not need to be long; indeed should *not* be long. Sleeping during the day means less kip at night.

Naps of 10–20 minutes are worth their weight in gold in terms of their restorative benefit and improved functioning on every level.

A survey by the National Institute for Occupational Safety and Health found they significantly improve alertness, mood and job performance. This is because the sleep that helps your body to recover and restore itself happens almost as soon as you fall asleep – which is why a nap is so powerful.

The ideal time to nap is, predictably, between 1 and 3 p.m., corresponding to the natural dip in our body clock which triggers sleepiness. Naps are for the day: generally, if you're after better sleep, nightime naps won't do the job.

There is one occasion, however, where you would be advised *not* to nap: if you are trying sleep-restriction therapy (see page 200).

Can't nap, won't nap

Many chronic insomniacs, myself included, simply can't nap, however tired we are. The official view is that we are insufficiently sleep-deprived. You decide. It feels pretty deprived to me.

A kinder interpretation is that, though it doesn't feel like it to us, we're hyper-aroused and spend most of our time on red alert, so that whatever is keeping us awake at night is also keeping us awake during the day. Another theory is that because we're awash with anxiety and worry about sleep (or whatever else is on our mind), the minute we have nothing to distract us and try and be still, this comes to the fore, preventing us from napping. The tips and information later in this book can help with this.

Dream on

Dreams and dreaming are profoundly important. As experts explain, dreams shine symbolic spotlights on your waking life, enabling you to access your intuitive wisdom and gain new insights into what you really need and want. They thus increase your potential for self-awareness and well-being. For Sigmund Freud, they were the 'royal road to the unconscious'. For Carl Jung, who worked with the inner processes and dynamics revealed by dreams,

z z z z

they were as much about memories collected since time began, which he termed the 'collective unconscious'.

Though it doesn't seem or feel so, we are not mere onlookers but the playwrights and stage-managers of our dreams (you can even ask yourself to dream a solution to whichever dilemma is currently keeping you awake), and understanding them is to be encouraged. Writing them down is a good first step – however bizarre they seem at first, you will find patterns emerging that soon start to make sense. If you find this useful, think about getting some expert advice on how to map and interpret your dreams: they could hold important clues about what's causing your insomnia, and may even help you to solve it.

For insomniacs, dreams fulfil another important role. Often they're the only sure sign we've been asleep. This is the other reason I try so hard to remember dreams every time I wake up – and would encourage every insomniac, or anyone who is not sleeping well, to do likewise. A dream can't offer the same relief as a sleeping pill, but it can be a life-line. Put simply, if you've dreamed, you've slept; and if you've slept once, you can sleep again. Holding on to your last dream as a 'hook' to help you get back to sleep is a good tip.

Many people say they don't dream: this is not so, they just don't remember them. In normal sleepers, for example, dreams add up to about 100 minutes' worth a night. If you make a conscious effort to remember your dreams, they will soon start tumbling out. Looking forward to the opportunity to dream, and viewing sleep like a movie – a pleasurable interlude of escapism which you can indulge in nightly – is a very good idea. It shifts the burden and anxiety of getting yourself to sleep (negative) into the delicious anticipation of seeing what tonight's dreamscape will offer. Which is a much nicer way to view your sleep, and much more fun.

Not everyone agrees with the symbolic importance attached to dreams – for a reasoned and scientific overview of what dreams are and what they might do, take a look at Professor Jim Horne's articles at http/sleep.lboro.ac.uk, under 'recent articles'.

What regulates sleep?

Sleep is the ultimate body–mind phenomenon, and what regulates, and hence disturbs, sleep is as complex as the nature of sleep itself. The potent cocktail of genes, proteins, hormones and neurotransmitters that control sleep is still being discovered. Physical, mental, emotional, social and external factors all play their part. This chapter explores the four prime biological regulators of sleep: body bio-rhythms, light, temperature and sleep promoting/regulating hormones.

Stress hormones and stimulants, the other two major drivers that adversely affect sleep, are discussed on pages 31 and 38. The role played by diet is discussed on page 107.

Nature's time-keeper: your body clock

Brain waves shape your sleep, but it is your internal body clock-cum-pacemaker that programmes you for sleep in the first place.

Everything in nature is conditioned by regular cycles or bio-rhythms of one sort or another, of which the daily 24-hour cycle of the sun, and seasonal cycles, are two of the most important. We are no exception: our bio-rhythms determine how well we work, rest and play – and much else besides.

The human daily rhythm is a 25-hour cycle – hence its name, 'circadian rhythm' from the Latin *circa diem*, 'about a day'. Irrespective of how much sleep we have or haven't had the night

zzzz

before, our bodies are internally set to experience two natural periods of sleepiness during any 24- to 25-hour period. It's this innate pre-programmed pacemaker that sets the timing for your own sleep pattern. It's what causes jet-lag, and why shift-work is usually a struggle.

Whether we like it or not, we are thus programmed to fall asleep at night, when it's dark and cooler (and, from an evolutionary perspective, safer), and to be awake when it's light and relatively warmer. Midnight – 7 a.m. is prime bodyclock sleep-time. The second sleep-spell we are programmed for is in mid-afternoon (1–3 p.m.). Which means the desire to nap or take a siesta after lunch is perfectly natural.

In the real world, however, life isn't that neat. Though everybody's personal pacemaker is set slightly differently, sleepwise, the world divides into two broad types – and knowing which you are, or tend towards, is critical to understanding your own sleep (and therefore lack of sleep) patterns.

Owls

Owls are those of us whose internal clocks run slightly slower than 24 hours and whose daily cycle is therefore slightly longer – perhaps as long as 28 hours in extreme cases. This is known as *phase-delay*. As a consequence, owls naturally want to go to bed late, get up late, are slow to get going in the morning and generally not good to be around first thing, but come into their own in the evening.

Owls often have more difficulty getting to sleep and may stay in light sleep longer, and the fact that they are so groggy when the time comes to wake up is because they are probably still in relatively deep sleep. An owl's circadian cycle may begin at around 9 a.m., and not finish until 1 a.m. If owls go to bed too early, they spend a long time getting to sleep; if they get up too early, they feel like they haven't had enough sleep. Staying in bed in the morning exacerbates the problem, as this delays the normal speeding-up of the clock, which is triggered by early morning light.

What's all the fuss about?

z z z z

Larks

Larks are those of us whose internal clock runs slightly faster than 24 hours and whose daily cycle is therefore slightly shorter – as little as 21 hours in extreme cases. This is known as *phase-advance*. As a consequence, larks naturally want to go to bed early, get up early, are bright and bushy-tailed the minute they get up, but become dormice in the evening. Larks tend to fall asleep easily and reach deep sleep quickly. A lark's circadian cycle may begin at 7 a.m. and finish at 9 p.m. Larks could force themselves to stay up later, but are still likely to wake up early. Numerically, larks predominate.

From a sleep-management viewpoint, it's easy to see that understanding the confines of your bodyclock is crucial. There's little point, for example, telling insomniac larks like me to stay up into the early hours of the morning, or expect insomniac owls to go to bed early when all they will do is thrash around even longer. As Professor Chris Idzikowski wisely says in *Sleep Well*, ideally it's more productive to allow your biological clock to dictate the amount of time you spend asleep, whilst you concentrate on improving the quality of that sleep. As he also points out, being an owl or a lark doesn't necessarily mean you're an insomniac – lots of people I've talked to clearly sleep pretty well, it's just that their bodyclocks aren't quite in tune with the 'norm'.

Your circadian rhythm – and hence your ability to sleep – changes with time. Generally we can expect to become more owl-like during adolescence, and more lark-like as we get older. Jet-lag and shift-work are the two examples par excellence of temporarily disrupted circadian rhythms.

Disorientated bodyclocks are a feature of insomnia generally; sleep-restriction therapy (page 200) is an effective way of helping to re-set it. More serious circadian rhythm disorders, such as Delayed Sleep Phase Syndrome (extreme owl-like) or Advanced Sleep Phase Syndrome (extreme lark-like) behaviours are classified as sleep disorders, and are thought to be genetically linked; which is why sleep disturbance can run in families. For more on these, see page 194.

z z z z

Sleep vs wakefulness

As well as the push and pull of your circadian rhythm, the brain has its own sleep and wakefulness centres tussling with each other. The sleep centre is located in the same region that is involved with body temperature, quite close to the bodyclock centre, the suprachiasmatic nucleus (SCN), discussed below. The wakefulness centre is located further down, in the brain stem region. Predictably, good sleepers have strong daytime wakefulness and night-time sleep systems; those who do not have an awake system that is too strong and a sleep system that is too weak. Scientists now believe they have found the hormone that controls this, called orexin. (For more on this, see page 24.)

Whatever and wherever the mind is, it plays its own crucial part in sleep. If your bodyclock and sleep-wakefulness centres are not working properly, or are damaged in some way, you will not sleep; the same goes for a disturbed mind. Which came first is a bit of a moot point.

Light

Too few of us get enough natural sunlight these days. Sunlight boosts the production of the feel-good hormone, serotonin (see page 21) and oestrogen, and generally makes the world a happier, brighter place.

Daylight (and lack of it) is the all-important signal that governs sleep, regulating both the circadian rhythm and the production of the sleep hormone melatonin (see page 22).

Briefly, natural daylight triggers the bodyclock centre, the suprachiasmatic nucleus (SNC) to send signals to the pineal gland to stop producing melatonin. In the evening, when light fades, the opposite happens and the pineal gland is stimulated to increase production of melatonin. This helps to explain why we naturally sleep less well in summer, and tend to get sleepier in winter. And why larks love early winter nights, and owls hate them.

z z z z

Sunlight vs artificial light

Though we may spend our lives under artificial light, it doesn't begin to compare with the real stuff. Natural light is significantly brighter (and whiter) than artificial light, and infinitely more powerful. A bright day, for example, radiates 10–30,000 lux, a cloudy day 3–15,000 lux. A typical office will generate around 200–400 lux of artificial light, and evening light at home 10–100 lux. If you've ever wondered why gardeners and people who work outside are generally contented folks, this is part of the reason.

Temperature

Your body temperature plays as important a role as light in governing sleep. It, too, is conditioned by your bodyclock, and over the course of a day will rise and fall by about 1½ degrees Farenheit. It's lowest when you are asleep in the early morning hours (around 4 a.m. for many normal sleepers) and highest in the early evening, at around 6 p.m. Critically, the onset of sleep is triggered by a dip in body temperature.

We have all experienced being too hot in bed to sleep, or, as an insomniac, the relief when you start to feel yourself become cool, and then sleep follows. One of the difficulties for insomniacs is that our body temperature doesn't fluctuate as much as in normal sleepers. Body temperature patterns also change with age, mimicking changes in sleep patterns. Thus, in the elderly, daily variations are muted, and body temperatures start to rise and fall earlier – all of which leads to less sleep. This is exacerbated by lack of exercise – another common characteristic of insomniacs and the elderly. For women, hot flushes associated with the menopause, are another significant disrupter of sleep. Massaging your body temperature is a recognized sleep therapy, and is essentially why sleep experts advise taking exercise or having a hot bath at strategic times, which raise body temperature so it then falls again at bedtime.

The temperature of your environment also affects your body temperature, and can have a profound effect on your sleep. Though extremes – a freezing cold bedroom or a hot midsummer, sultry one – will both stop you sleeping, you will cool down much faster in bed if your bedroom is cool rather than hot. There'll be more on this on page 105.

Two important sleep organs: the SCN and the pineal gland

The SCN (suprachiasmatic nucleus) houses your bodyclock. It's made up of a pair of pinhead structures in the hypothalamus of the brain, positioned just above the point where the optic nerves cross, about 3 cm behind the eyes, and comprising a cluster of around 12–15,000 neurones. The SCN is sensitive to changes in light and temperature, helps synchronize sleep with the natural 24-hour cycle of day and night, and regulates a range of body functions which affect sleep, such as temperature, hormonal secretion and changes in blood pressure – and, crucially, directs the pineal gland to produce melatonin.

The story doesn't end there: the latest research is examining whether every cell in the body has the potential to be a bodyclock – and, if so, how they talk to each other.

The pineal gland, often called 'the third eye' – which indeed, being light sensitive, it is – is found towards the back of the top of the brain. It produces melatonin. Many living creatures possess one, including reptiles, for whom it is a true third eye. In addition to being a prime player in sleep, the pineal gland is also responsible for sexual development and helps regulate the immune system. According to Yogic philosophy, the pineal gland has a connection with *Ajna*, the mental or 'inner eye' chakra energy centre, and occupies approximately the same location in the brain. A troubled mind impacts negatively on the pineal gland, leading to impaired sleep.

z z z z

The biochemistry of sleep

A rudimentary appreciation of what's happening bio-chemically in the jigsaw called sleep can help us to understand the knock-on effects of upsetting nature's carefully prescribed levels of hormones in your body.

The role of serotonin and melatonin

Serotonin and melatonin are words that you may have heard bandied about. Both are natural hormones produced in the brain, and are the two vital chemicals associated with sleep. They are intimately linked – serotonin is the precursor of melatonin. Without enough of either, we don't sleep. It's as simple as that.

Serotonin

Serotonin is one of *the* most important brain chemicals. You need it to sleep and to be happy. Indeed, serotonin is our very own Prozac (Prozac and other anti-depressants are all specific serotonin-boosters). Lack of serotonin not only results in insomnia but also anxiety and depression – two of insomnia's most common bedfellows – and various mood disorders from panic attacks, irritability, anger, PMT, SAD (seasonal affective disorder) and more. People with low self-esteem or guilt complexes, or who worry or are obsessive (sound familiar?) often have low serotonin levels.

There is an important gender difference here, with men getting the better deal. Men produce serotonin twice as fast as women, which means they have the ability, generally, to recover from any shortfall more quickly. Women produce up to a third less than men: it seems we are programmed to be moody, which statistics confirm. In addition, low serotonin in women is associated with depression and anxiety; in men it's associated more with aggression and alcoholism. Add to this the fact that low oestrogen levels also result in low serotonin levels – see page 24 – and it's a wonder we ever feel chirpy.

Although serotonin is produced in the brain, around 90 per cent is found in the gut. It plays a role in appetite control, and if you suffer from carbohydrate cravings, this may indicate low serotonin levels. Your heart is also partly dependent on serotonin, so that lack of serotonin can affect both your digestion and your heart.

Serotonin is produced in the brain from tryptophan, one of the essential amino acids you need to take in via your diet (discussed in detail on page 115). Light affects its levels (more light, more serotonin). Exercise and oxygen also help to boost its production. A poor diet, alcohol, caffeine and the artificial sweetener aspartame all rob you of your precious serotonin, as does stress. This is because in an effort to keep you calm, your brain releases more serotonin, diverting its precious supplies to cope with the stress rather than to promote sleep. Apart from a lack of tryptophan, Patrick Holford in *Optimum Nutrition for the Mind,* identifies the main causes of serotonin deficiency as: lack of oestrogen (women) or testosterone (men), not enough light, not enough exercise, too much stress (especially for women) and finally, not enough co-factor vitamins and minerals.

Nor does it end there. As one sleep scientist explains, serotonin is talked about as if it were a simple neurotransmitter, when in fact it's a lot more complicated. It has at least 8–12 different receptors, with different associated control mechanisms. Simple increases and decreases in serotonin also have different effects on bodily systems. No wonder your sleep suffers. It's easy to see, too, how an insomniac quickly succumbs to other negative side-effects of an imbalance of serotonin – let alone whatever is happening with your melatonin and stress hormones.

The way out of this vicious circle is to try and boost your levels of serotonin, either by getting more exercise (page 137), getting more light (page 194), taking supplements (see page 124) or increasing the amount of tryptophan in your diet (see page 115). Psychologists offer an easier option: build in at least 30 minutes' worth of things that make you happy into your day.

Melatonin

Anyone who has insomnia or who has tried to alleviate jet-lag will have heard of melatonin, nature's soporific sleep-inducing hormone, produced in the tiny pineal gland at the base of the brain, and which was only discovered 50 years ago. Melatonin orchestrates sleep by preparing the body to sleep. As already discussed, its production is regulated by light (see page 18). It's produced at night, triggered by the fading light as the sun sets. When dawn comes, melatonin levels drop quickly, and are virtually undetectable during the day. Overnight urine contains a high concentration of melatonin, which is why some Indian Holy men drink it (to keep themselves calm). Not surprisingly, we produce more in winter than summer. A rise in melatonin signals a decrease in body temperature (which promotes sleep); a decrease in melatonin signals a rise in body temperature (wakefulness).

How much light affects melatonin production differs from person to person – for example, some people shut down production virtually immediately if exposed to unexpected bright light during the night; for others this takes up to an hour. Children produce most melatonin; this drops at puberty and wanes with age, dropping sharply at the onset of middle-age. Increasing your melatonin levels, usually by supplementation, is a well-known 'cure' for jet-lag and insomnia, and has also been hailed as a means of combating the ageing process, as it is a potent antioxidant and scavenger of free radicals, and a powerful immune system-enhancer. In short, we all need lots of lovely melatonin.

Melatonin is produced from serotonin. The only sure way to know whether you are making enough is to pay for a private saliva test (for details, see page 267). Caffeine, tobacco, alcohol, dark chocolate, certain drugs – aspirin, antidepressants and tranquillizers – and being close to electrical appliances will all rob you of melatonin.

There are four ways to try and boost melatonin levels (and hence improve your sleep):

1. using light to stimulate production (page 194)
2. taking melatonin supplements (page 127)
3. taking serotonin supplements (page 125)
4. increasing tryptophan (which converts to serotonin, which converts to melatonin) either in your diet or by taking supplements (pages 115 and 126).

z z z z

If you have jet-lag, for example, you can also use melatonin to help re-set your biological clock (see page 195). For the latest on melatonin, see www.smartlifenews.com.

Orexin

This is the latest discovery, hot from the research labs. Orexin is a brain neuropeptide, or more correctly a pair of hormones, Orexin A and B, produced in the hypothalamus, believed to control your wakefulness system. Put simply, at night your bodyclock stops the hypothalamus from producing orexin chemical, and hence we sleep. Looked at another way, orexin has the potential to keep you awake for 24 hours. It's been hailed as a potential cure for narcolepsy (narcoleptics produce far less orexin than normal people); the US Army is interested in using it to keep soldiers alert instead of amphetamines. For the rest of us, watch this space.

Orexin's other function is linked to appetite control; its name comes from the Greek *orexis*, for appetite. Some fantasize that one day we can use orexin or drugs to control it to be permanently slim and permanently awake – with no side-effects.

Women: a special case

Women are more prone to insomnia than men. In part, this is due to the effect of the female hormones oestrogen and progesterone. Oestrogen is needed to stimulate production of serotonin, and low oestrogen usually results in lower levels of serotonin. Low progesterone prevents the amino acid GABA (see page 129) from doing its job of making you relax. A sudden drop in progesterone, for example before your period, can result in the insomnia associated with PMS. Levels of both decline, sometimes spectacularly, during the menopause, which is when women often experience insomnia. Note that men can also suffer from low progesterone. (For more on women and serotonin, see page 21.)

Why *can't* we sleep?

The question that burns in every insomniac's brain. Nature may have equipped us with a wonderfully elegant solution for taking a break from the toil of everyday life – 'nature's soft purse', as Shakespeare describes it in *Henry IV* – but the reality is that this 'solution' doesn't always seem to function half as well as it should. The reason for this is that not being able to sleep well is rarely due to a single cause, but to a web of circumstances that often tangle themselves into complicated knots to form the well-known vicious circle we call insomnia. It's unpicking this mess, and teasing it out thread by thread, that you have to do to understand your insomnia.

The 'causes' or initial reasons why we find ourselves having difficulty in sleeping vary from the mildly irritating – dogs barking in the night – to unexpected traumas, grief such as bereavement and, most frustrating of all for many of us, free-floating anxiety of all kinds. It may be caused by medical illnesses, or various physical sleep disorders such as sleep apnoea. Psychological and emotional issues are other obvious causes. Certain drugs will also cause insomnia. Lifestyle factors that severely disrupt sleep include a poor diet and snoring partners. Many of these you can easily do something about – and should do. We'll take a close look at how to get started in Part 3.

z z z z

Check It Out

Here is a quick A–Z of the main factors that contribute to poor sleep and insomnia:

Age

As we get older, getting less sleep and changing sleep patterns are facts of life. You can learn to adjust by adopting good sleep habits and positive behavioural tactics (see page 179).

Anxiety

Anxiety is that vague constant feeling of apprehension, worry and non-specific general fear. Along with stress, it's one of the most common causes of insomnia. Because of its nature, it can be the trickiest to deal with, requiring much patience, tlc, creative mind games and an eclectic tool-bag full of things to help.

Babies (and children)

Unavoidably, new arrivals disrupt both parents' sleep. The importance of teaching your children good sleep habits is now becoming recognized. It's a serious issue for most parents. Look at www.amazon.com or www.amazon.co.uk and you will find that books on getting your baby to sleep feature prominently. The National Childbirth Trust's *Help Your Baby to Sleep* by Penny Hames is one good place to start. Baby massage and aromatherapy can help, too (see page 159).

Circadian rhythm disorders

This is a medical condition which means your circadian rhythms, and therefore your sleep, is out of synch. You either become an exaggerated owl or lark, or your bodyclock is on a permanent go-slow. If you suspect this is at the root of your insomnia, you need to seek specialist help. Bright Light therapy (page 194) is the treatment most commonly recommended.

What's all the fuss about?

z z z z

Drugs

Many drugs, including some you wouldn't expect such as over-the-counter medicines for asthma, colds and weight-loss, as well as steroids and beta-blockers, can disrupt sleep; some, including over-use of sleeping pills, can result in insomnia. So, too, do hard and soft drugs (marijuana can send some people off to sleep, but can equally disrupt it for others). If you are taking prescription drugs and you develop insomnia, check with your doctor to see if the drugs could be a cause.

Emotional factors

General emotional turbulence, negative or positive, about anything and everything from the trivial to the awesomely life-changing, can disturb sleep. It all depends on how acute the problem is. See Part 3, page 93, and start with the easy and obvious things first.

External environmental factors

Noise, TVs and computers in the bedroom, bed in the wrong place, the wrong bed, the wrong pillow and all the other little things such as bedroom curtains that let in too much light – all of these contribute to what sleep scientists call 'poor sleep hygiene'. Everyone can improve this. For more see page 101.

Food and drink

These matter more than you think – not just what you eat and drink, but when and how much. See Eating to Sleep (page 107) and The Terrible Trio (page 38).

Hormonal imbalance

Puberty, PMS and the menopause are three obvious examples, but any kind of serious hormonal imbalance or malfunctioning hormone-producing gland does not bode well for sleep, so you may want to get them checked out. This can often be done by a Traditional Chinese Medicine practitioner, naturopath, chiropractor, your family doctor or by private tests. An underactive thyroid (hypothyroidism), for example, affects the production of serotonin and melatonin, and an overactive one (hyperthyroidism) can make you hyper. For more on hormones and hormonal imbalances, see What Regulates Sleep (page 15) and Stress and Anxiety (page 31).

Lifestyle factors

It will not come as news to you that these can include erratic sleep habits, work habits, shift-work, working too hard, no exercise and eating and drinking all the wrong things. With the exception of work these hurdles to sleep are easy to solve, and we'll discuss them in more detail later in this book.

Medical illness

Any illness that causes discomfort, pain, indigestion, breathlessness or bladder problems can disrupt your sleep; if left unchecked this can lead to insomnia. If the illness is temporary, the insomnia is likely to be short term. Too many people, however – like Nick (see page 70) – are insomniacs because they developed the habit of not sleeping when they were ill.

Mental illness

It is a clinical fact that insomniacs often suffer depression, and depressives often suffer insomnia. Other psychological and psychiatric problems can also cause insomnia.

Sleep disorders

Over 80 different physical sleep disorders have been diagnosed. Most, such as serious snoring and sleep apnoea (when you block air waves for a microsecond some hundreds of times per night), are respiratory problems. Other disorders include narcolepsy (the frightening habit of falling asleep at the drop of a hat, which can be life-threatening), restless legs and periodic limb movement syndrome.

The majority of these, including sleep apnoea, are treatable, usually in sleep clinics. If you suspect some unheard-of sleeping disorder could be the cause of your sleeping problems, check it out with your doctor. For more on sleep clinics, see page 189.

z z z z

Social factors

Snoring partners, crying babies and restless children are all-too-common examples. It is not your fault, but only you can find a compromise which works in your household before you end up with a sleeping problem that won't go away, causing the whole family to suffer, not just you. The same goes for noisy flatmates – if you can't reach some kind of compromise, you need to move. For more, see Sleeping Partners (page 79).

Stimulants

For which read alcohol, caffeine and nicotine – the bad boys of sleep. All qualify as drugs. Alcoholics often suffer insomnia; once the alcohol dependency has been removed, it may still take some time for normal sleep patterns to return. At the risk of rubbing it in, see The Terrible Trio (page 38).

Stress

Another very common cause of insomnia. Stress is not the same as throwing an emotional wobbly, or being anxious. Stress is serious stuff, and if you have it, you won't get very far with resolving your insomnia until you acknowledge that stress is involved somewhere. For more, see Stress and Anxiety (page 31).

Temperature

Sleeping in an environment that's either too hot or too cold, or being too hot or cold, will keep you awake. For more, see What Regulates Sleep? (page 15) and Getting It Sorted (begins on page 93).

Wide-awake brain

Our old friend, being 'hyper-aroused' – having a brain that refuses to go away and behave itself so you can get some rest and deep sleep – is what many sleepless people do best, including myself. There is no statutory cure for this. Head for behavioural and relaxation therapies, and anyone who promises to take the fire out of your head. Or take the plunge and learn meditation. For more on this, and how insomniacs' sleep differs from that of normal sleepers, see Part 2, page 61, and Part 3, page 146.

z z z z

Women

Alas, we are a special case. Just about every study shows that women suffer more disturbed sleep than men. As well as the hormonal fluctuations already mentioned, insomnia is also common during the later stages of pregnancy. For more on our hormones see What Regulates Sleep? (page 15).

Insomnia as 'out of balance'

Pick up any book on Chinese or Ayurvedic medicine, or talk to any complementary health practitioner – be it a naturopath, homoeopath, chiropractor, reflexologist, kinesiologist, reiki specialist or any other practitioner who works with energy medicine, or any spiritual healer – and they all say the same thing. The holistic interpretation of insomnia is that you are not whole; that your body/mind/spirit balance is out of synch. The issue is how out of balance it might be, and why.

Chinese Traditional Medicine, for example, views insomnia as a symptom of weak heart energy. The heart is part of the Fire element, houses *Shen*, or spirit, and is symbolically associated with love, health and vitality. As Dr Jennifer Harper explains in *Nine Ways to Body Wisdom*, the heart affects our mental and emotional health. A weak heart signifies insomnia, poor memory, anxiety and low self-esteem.

In traditional Ayurvedic medicine, illness represents an imbalance of your dosha; insomnia signals too much air (*vata*) energy. For more, see Part 2, page 54 and the Complementary Therapies section of Part 4, beginning on page 211.

When should we start to worry?

Most people in the world experience the occasional bout of insomnia. A few nights of not sleeping well is OK, and something we all go through. A regular pattern of disrupted or bad sleep is not. Once you start to worry about it, then it's time for action.

z z z z

Acknowledging your insomnia early, and resolving to do something about it as THE TOP PRIORITY in your life, is the first and most important step you can take to help yourself.

Stress and anxiety

This may be an obvious thing to say, but stress is the most common reason for not being able to sleep. As sleep experts confirm, the two are inextricably linked: stress is a powerful disrupter of sleep, and insomnia is one of the first signs of stress. This is not good news when we live in a world where stress levels increase daily.

You can look at stress two ways. When we think of stress, we think of stress at work, family stress, the meeting-deadlines-being-too-busy-stress, and emotional and psychological stress. In other words, life-issues stress and the stress posed by the demands of everyday life.

Biologically, too, stresses that we don't give a second thought to, such as environmental pollutions, toxic overload – for instance, pesticide residues, junk diets, and stimulants like caffeine and nicotine (see page 38) – play their part. Allergies, too much exercise (to understand the highs and lows of the stress hormone adrenaline, try running a marathon) and chronic infections such as the flu are also all extremely stressful as far as your body is concerned. Looked at this way, it's a wonder any of us sleeps well, and you could argue that insomniacs are nearer 'normal' than others who sleep OK. Certainly, statistics on people who experience insomnia or regular disturbed sleep show that more and more of us are heading that way.

The problem is that, biologically, we are still in the stone age. For our body systems, stress means danger – i.e., short-term fear/flight/fight stress – and our bodies react the way they always have: with high levels of the stress hormones adrenaline and cortisol. We are simply not equipped to deal with the steady drip-drip, prolonged, sustained or cumulative stress that is so characteristic of modern life.

Both adrenaline and cortisol are produced in the adrenal glands – your body's hormone workhorses, situated on top of your kidneys.

A short burst of adrenaline puts your body on red alert, generating extra physical and mental energy so you can fight or flee. Adrenaline's effects are short-term. Cortisol, dubbed the 'can do' hormone, takes over and gives you the stamina and willpower to see the danger through. Put simply, adrenaline arms you to fight, and cortisol helps you win the battle.

So far, so good. Except it isn't. Though a certain amount of stress is fine – biologists even think it's good for you, as it helps you get away from the dinosaur faster than the chilled-out guy next to you – persistent or excessive stress is not. To say it affects your sleep and can induce insomnia is obvious. Stress depletes serotonin, melatonin and the relaxing hormone GABA (see page 129), so you get a double whammy: you can't sleep because you're stressed and you can't relax because the feel-good relaxing hormones are being thrashed. Stress during the day spills out into the night, over-activating the arousal system in the brain and elevating stress hormones which then remain elevated throughout the night, compounding the problem further – not least because high cortisol can elevate glucose levels in the blood by about 50 per cent, itself a recipe for disturbed sleep. Not surprisingly, stress reduces the amount of deep sleep you get, making the sleep you do get lighter and more unsatisfactory.

Even when the stress has gone away, cortisol levels can remain elevated. Cortisol levels are normally at their lowest late in the evening and into the night, but insomniacs often have high levels of cortisol in the evening – it is any wonder, then, that we don't sleep?

Equally worrying is that having your system awash with adrenaline and cortisol most of the time literally exhausts you and has a knock-on effect of contributing to illnesses such as heart disease, impaired memory and Alzheimer's disease (it can destroy the brain cells responsible for memory). It can also compromise your immune system. Because energy is being redirected to flee or fight, it is taken away from your digestive system and your repair and maintenance systems, which can lead to digestive problems and speeds up the ageing process. Eventually the adrenals start to wear out and become incapable of producing the required amount of hormones. When you get to the stage that insomniacs recognize well, where you have lost the plot completely, are overwhelmed by the simplest of tasks and can't face doing anything, your cortisol levels are likely to be rock-bottom.

This is why turning this one around is so important. It's probably the thing that will help get your sleep pattern back on track faster than anything else.

Thankfully, it's easier to take the pressure off your stress than you think. If you follow the steps outlined in Part 3, your stress levels *will* come down, and you *will* feel better for it.

Blood types and stress

A useful snippet, which fits me, and may fit you. According to Dr Peter J D'Adamo (see www.dadamo.com), those with blood type A can tolerate adrenaline better than those with blood type O; whilst those with blood type O can tolerate cortisol better than those with blood type A. (Note that, with respect to stress, blood type B tends to be like blood type A, while blood type AB tends to be like blood type O.) This means that people with blood type A, like me, are better at dealing with short-term panics than people with blood type O, who tend to get agitated very quickly, but are less able than those with blood type O to cope with sustained pressure – anxiety disorders are thus more prevalent, due likely to high cortisol and possibly low melatonin levels. In these cases, blood group specialists suggest treatment that focuses on cortisol rather than serotonin imbalance (St John's Wort/Prozac, etc.). It also means that those with type A need the kind of exercise or disciplines that will soothe away the cortisol and calm them, such as yoga, Tai Chi, or meditation, whilst those with type O are generally better with high-energy sports such as running to flush the adrenaline out of their system.

Those with blood type O also have lower levels of monoamine oxidase (MAO), which metabolizes the hormones dopamine and adrenaline; depression is also more prevalent among those with blood type O. As we've seen, insomnia and depression often go hand in hand. MAO-inhibitor antidepressant drugs (MAOIs) are thus *not* recommended for people with blood type O. This includes St John's Wort and Kava-kava.

To get your blood group analysed, see page 267.

A note on anxiety

Stress is different from anxiety. Stress is a physiological response, whereas anxiety is behavioural in origin. Anxiety can cause stress, which is why if you are anxious you are likely to be stressed. Maria (see page 36) is a classic case of an insomniac who is anxious rather than stressed, but whose anxiety, when it gets bad, causes her stress. Learning to stop being anxious about your insomnia, therefore, will automatically reduce your stress levels.

Anxiety, depression and insomnia

A bleak thought indeed, but anxiety, depression and insomnia are natural bedfellows. People who are anxious or depressed often experience insomnia. This is why, if you go and see your family doctor about your insomnia, he or she will usually ask you first if you are depressed. This is also why doctors often prescribe anti-depressants as first-line treatment for insomnia.

Insomniacs are inevitably anxious (at least about their sleep) and often develop depression. From a sleep scientist's perspective, not being able to get to sleep and waking up frequently (onset and maintenance insomnia) are often associated with anxiety, whilst waking up frequently and waking up early are often associated with depression.

Depression

Depression is a continuum of feelings that range from feeling down and a bit bleak, apathetic or sad, in its mild form, to that underworld of worthlessness and state of absolute downheartedness and nothingness where anything is too much trouble and everything is too much effort. Psychiatrists also describe it as anger turned inwards, pointing out that many people become depressed because they are betraying themselves in some way.

Everyone gets depressed sometimes. Experiencing some form of depression because you have insomnia or are sleeping badly is

z z z z

pretty common, too. For some, like myself, it can get more serious for a time, and it's worth being aware of this so you can nip it in the bud before it becomes part of your emerging sleep-deprived *alter ego*.

However many causes depression may have, it is also a function of brain chemistry. The 'chemical blues', as nutritionist Patrick Holford describes it, is a result of low serotonin (mood hormone) and adrenaline and noradrenaline (motivation hormones). As already described, the link with insomnia becomes obvious, especially for women.

Insomnia and burnout

Three-quarters through writing this book I was given a book called *The Joy of Burnout* by Dr Dina Glouberman. The book shook me rigid, for it seemed to be an accurate account of how I felt about my insomnia and my life. Burnout is most commonly associated with work, but is equally applicable to other areas of your life. The term describes the symptoms well – exhaustion on every level, often accompanied by illness. Insomnia is a common symptom, as are loss of appetite, depression, anxiety, anger, emotional deadness, isolation and poor attention. These symptoms, however, are merely the tip of the pyramid of burnout. The real cause and meaning lie much deeper.

Often confused with mid-life crisis, which can be a form of burnout, burnout is an underlying, deeply felt malaise and fundamental crisis in your life. Dr Glouberman describes it as a state of mind, body and spirit reached by those who have come to the end of a particular road but who haven't acknowledged it – the result of having become better able to hear our souls but not yet daring to listen to them. As she explains, burnout demands that you listen. If your insomnia is a symptom of burnout, it may be your body/mind/spirit's way of forcing you to do so. It is, quite literally, the wake-up call of your life.

Burnout is a tough call. It takes time for the penny to drop, and even when it does, it's much easier to look away. But it is also a path to liberation. The liberation may be modest or profoundly life-changing (and challenging), but one thing is certain: You will never

zzzz

be quite the same again. How many insomniacs this applies to is impossible to ascertain, but if you have an inkling that this might be behind your insomnia, getting better at managing it by using the various means and suggestions in this book is just part of what you need to do. For lasting relief, you will need to confront your version of burnout. You may also, as I did, need to acknowledge the unthinkable: that you yourself are nurturing and promoting your insomnia; that however crazy it may seem, you want it in your life. Once it stops being useful, you can let go and the cure can begin in earnest.

Typical candidates for burnout are high-energy, ambitious and capable achievers; we need to be needed, approved of and feel special in some way; we often overdo and, especially, over-give. During burnout, in some ways, we could be called *un*-hearted rather than *whole*-hearted, in the sense of feeling empty or of not being touched by things that usually make our hearts sing, and that despite what we may think and others who know us think, we are disconnected from ourselves. Reading *The Joy of Burnout* will help you decide whether you're a candidate – or whether you can breathe a sigh of relief and are just plain exhausted.

Crying works

Crying is a natural reaction to stress. Like other people I know, when things would get really bad in the middle of a sleepless night I would have two urges: to scream and to cry. Screaming is a bit impractical, so I cried instead.

Crying is good. Human tears contain adrenocorticotrophic hormone (ACTH), responsible for initiating the stress response. When you cry, you wash this hormone away.

Maria's story – the hyper-anxious insomniac

We are constantly being told that not being able to sleep is 'all in the mind'. This may be largely true, but nevertheless it seems that some

z z z z

of us are primarily victims of our own cock-eyed biochemistry. This was certainly the case of Maria, 37, a reflexologist and one of the nicest people you could wish to meet.

My anxiety and consequent insomnia have ruled my life for eight years now, since I was 29, when depression hit me out of the blue. It's cyclical. I can be fine, and sleep fine, for a few weeks, then it kicks in. The insomnia is full-on – I can't eat, have panic attacks, and I become hyper-anxious about anything and everything. I look at that other person I have become and know I don't want this, and don't need it, but am powerless to do anything about it. I've tried everything – antidepressants, tranquillizers, St John's Wort – you name it, I've tried it.

The stress and anxiety feed each other. It's a vicious roller-coaster of discontentment and of driving yourself even harder. It disables you. You worry about the worry and have a deep-rooted fear of fear. I don't understand why I go into it any more than I know how or why I pull out of it. As far as the insomnia is concerned, I will try anything anyone tells me – nothing yet has worked. With me, sleep happens when it wants to happen, not when I read a book, play tapes or do any of that. Even sleeping pills only knock me out for an hour or so. I will fall asleep exhausted on the sofa, wake up totally disorientated, don't even wash my face but get straight into bed – and my brain says, 'Ding. You're not going anywhere.' I can then lie awake until about 4 a.m. and then grab a couple of hours until the alarm rings at 6. No two nights are ever the same. People tell me I should get up but I'm frightened that will make me more awake, and anyway I prefer to stay in bed.

All the time I'm holding down a job, and no one, unless they know me really well, has a clue at what I'm going through. The bouts usually last 2–3 weeks, sometimes longer, then my body literally gives up. I crash out and get a good night's sleep, and my sleep will then be reasonable until something throws it (or me) again. I deal with it because it's patchy – it's the one comfort I have. It's also probably why I haven't bothered trying to find a long-term cure that works for me, even though it rules my life.

Being pregnant has changed all of this: For the first time I feel calm, at peace with myself, and am sleeping much better. I'm convinced it has to be a hormonal imbalance. However, I can't quite believe it's over. As far as I'm concerned I'm still an insomniac.

The terrible trio: caffeine, alcohol and nicotine

Ironically, the world's three most favourite pastimes – drinking coffee and alcohol, and smoking – are all anathema to good sleep. In the sleep business, they're known as 'sleep thieves'. Which makes life very boring for insomniacs.

Caffeine

Caffeine is the world's most favourite stimulant. Found in over 60 plants worldwide, we consume vast quantities of it daily in coffee, tea, colas and other soft carbonated drinks. Guarana is also high in caffeine, though unless you drink organic soft drinks, or go to Brazil, you probably won't have heard of it. Just over half is drunk as coffee. It's also found in some pain relievers, cold and flu remedies and appetite suppressants (dieting aids), and in certain foods, notably cocoa and chocolate. It's also addictive, which is why it is often described as the world's favourite drug.

Caffeine is a very effective wake-up tool, which is why we feel so good – and alert – when we drink it. It is readily absorbed, in as little as 15–30 minutes, though its effects last 3–4 hours or longer (some estimates say up to 12 hours).

Caffeine has a powerful effect on the brain, and levels in the brain mimic that in the body, except that large doses can remain in the brain for 9–15 hours. Caffeine stimulates the central nervous system (brain and spinal cord), increasing metabolic, blood pressure, heart and breathing rates, and induces pleasurable feel-good mood changes in the brain.

As insomniacs know, it's the drug of choice to offset sleep-deprivation. This is not a good idea. Where sleep is concerned, chemically, caffeine packs a triple whammy. At a molecular level, caffeine is similar to adenosine, an important natural sedative found in the brain. Caffeine blocks the effects of adenosine, and it's this action that denies us the relaxing benefits of adenosine and keeps us alert. Because it's also a stimulant, it excites your nerves, which causes your pituitary gland to release another shot of adrenaline. And, thirdly, caffeine lowers melatonin levels.

An intake of 300+ mg of caffeine is thought to reduce REM sleep, and causes you to wake up more often. Drinking caffeine around bedtime, or even after lunchtime, is a definite no-no. It increases the time it takes to get to sleep, the amount you toss and turn and how often you wake up, and decreases the amount of deep sleep you get and how long you sleep for.

Being a perpetual kill-joy is rotten. As most people get their caffeine fix through drinking coffee, it's worth pointing out that coffee at least has some redeeming features that neither alcohol (except for red wine) nor nicotine can boast. It's high in antioxidants, its alertness and mood-enhancing properties means that it enables you to perform better, albeit on a temporary basis, and it is classed as a beneficial food for blood type A individuals.

How much caffeine?

Medical doctors disagree on how much caffeine is good or bad for you. Most health practitioners advise keeping off the stuff entirely. Like chilli, everyone's sensitivity to it varies. This is because some people are better at metabolizing it than others; the slower you metabolize it, the longer it and its effects remains in your system. Note that contraceptive pills slow down its elimination, and that caffeine remains in the system 2–7 times longer during late pregnancy: there are no placental barriers to it, so the foetus is exposed to its effects. Heredity plays its part, which is maybe why we need to be weaned onto the stuff while South Americans apparently don't. Like chilli, too, the more you have, the more you can tolerate. Tea and coffee are the main culprits, followed by canned drinks. Unless I've got my sums wrong, chocolate does not pose a caffeine problem for sleep (unless you're a serious chocaholic) – though don't have it after dinner or before bedtime.

The orthodox medical view is that a moderate consumption of 250 mg per day – about 2 150-ml cups of ground roasted coffee, or $1^1/2$ shots of espresso – is reckoned to pose no harm, nor is it linked to serious illnesses such as heart disease or cancer. All fine, except it's actually very difficult to determine your precise caffeine intake – the caffeine content of coffee, for example, varies according to the type. Real coffee, for example, has twice that of instant coffee. It's the same with tea, which despite its image actually contains substantial amounts of caffeine. Strong tea is not far short of instant coffee; the figure usually given is 40–60 mg of caffeine per cup of tea, and 65 mg per cup of instant coffee. Published figures also vary.

Still feel like persisting? The National Sleep Foundation in the USA has its own helpful caffeine calculator on its website: www.sleepfoundation.org/caffeine.html.

Caffeine Ready Reckoner
A rough rule of thumb:

1 cup filtered coffee	100 mg
1 cup instant coffee	66 mg
1 cup decaff	3 mg
1 cup tea (tea bag)	40 mg

Note: It depends how long you brew tea for; the darker the brew, the more the caffeine. Figures for brewed tea range from 60–180 mg.

1 cup tea (loose tea)	41 mg
1 cup green tea	4 mg
1 can energy drink	80 mg
1 can cola (regular or diet)	23 mg

Note: Other figures put this higher: 37 mg for regular cola, 46 mg for diet cola.

50-gm bar of plain chocolate	20–32 mg
50-gm bar of milk chocolate	7–9 mg
1 cup hot chocolate	5 mg
1 cup cocoa	15 mg

Source: Various, including *The Food and Mood Handbook*.

---

z z z z

What's all the fuss about?

Alcohol

People who drink are adamant that alcohol puts them to sleep. It does, because it's a sedative, but it then wakes you up again (this is known as 'rebound wakefulness'), and has just as disruptive an effect on sleep as caffeine.

A little is OK, but the habit of drinking to zonk you out so you can sleep doesn't work. Chemically, it causes the release of adrenaline and blocks tryptophan (see page 115) from getting to the brain. Even when there is no alcohol left in your system, it affects sleep patterns adversely. If pregnant women drink it can affect the sleep patterns of the foetus – this is one of the reasons women are advised not to drink during pregnancy. It's thought particularly to reduce REM sleep in the second half of the night, as well as deep sleep, and you are likely to feel knackered the next day. It's also a diuretic, which means you will need to get up in the night to pee, and impairs breathing, so can exacerbate snoring.

Alcohol abuse and alcoholism often result in insomnia; and alcoholism is twice as common in insomniacs as in normal sleepers.

One unit of alcohol (half a pint of beer, 1 glass of wine) takes about 1 hour to metabolize. So if you drink 3 glasses of wine at 10 p.m., expect your sleep to be disrupted from around 1 a.m.

All this needs to be set in context. For example, the medical profession doesn't seem to distinguish between wine, beer or spirits, nor their different effects physically and emotionally, nor the social circumstances under which you consume the alcohol. It all depends, too, on your particular threshold and ability to metabolize alcohol. Men can tolerate more than women, for example. (Winston Churchill famously had brandy for breakfast, and drank a bottle of champagne at lunch and dinner every night.)

Wine enthusiasts (I'm married to one) argue vigorously that a glass or two of red wine taken with your meal, and in a leisurely, contemplative way, will aid sleep, and will not necessarily wake you up either. That's decent wine, not plonk. This is not an excuse to drink a bottle and to blame me when you are awake in the middle of the night. Merely food for thought. How many wine enthusiasts would sleep better without their beloved wine? I don't know. Mine wouldn't even countenance the thought.

Nicotine

Nicotine is as lethal as caffeine and alcohol for disrupting your sleep: the average smoker takes twice as long to fall asleep as a non-smoker, and sleeps 30 minutes less, producing the same unwelcome effects as listed above for caffeine. Nictoine's relaxing properties are short-lived, and more to due with its addictive nature (you've satisfied your craving and therefore feel relaxed). Like caffeine, it's a powerful stimulant (it mimics acetylcholine, one of the three key activating neurotransmitters), and triggers the release of the 'fight or flight' hormone, adrenaline.

Recently it has been discovered that nicotine acts like cocaine in the brain by stimulating a second key neurotransmitter, dopamine, which triggers pleasure. Like alcohol, once metabolized, nicotine wakes you up.

The more you smoke, the worse the effects. When people give up smoking, though this is not always the case, their sleep may suffer more, temporarily, due to withdrawal symptoms, but then improves.

For more on these three, see page 110.

What happens
when we don't get
enough sleep?

When I first started delving into insomnia, I frightened myself to bits – and made my insomnia much worse – by reading about all the ills I was likely to develop through lack of sleep. The good – or, should I say, official news – is that although lack of sleep can be debilitating in the extreme and is a profoundly disagreeable condition to have to live with, persistent lack of sleep does not cause major illness. It does, however, cause a series of very unpleasant symptoms and side-effects, which if not addressed will make your life miserable and lead to severe mental, emotional and physical stress – which is the real killer.

The daily effects of insomnia are predictable and well known: daytime fatigue, irritability, anxiety, impaired concentration and decreased alertness. How well you cope with these depends on recognizing them for what they are – side-effects – and being able to get to grips with them. In Part 3 (beginning on page 93) you'll see how to get started. For now, a few points on these pesky side-effects:

Anxiety: Being anxious is a state of mind, a feeling of fear, apprehension or worry, an internal ever-present background noise, where the volume gets turned up or down depending on the circumstances. Some of us, myself included, are just made this way, and if you are the anxious type you are likely to be a poor sleeper. It's natural to feel anxious about insomnia, but you also need to work out whether it's the insomnia or you. Believe me, it can help a lot. For the difference between stress and anxiety, see page 31.

z z z z

Being normal: No book mentions this, but it is a fact that once insomnia bites hard you don't feel normal or like 'you'. For more on this, see page 70.

Being rational: Sleep deprivation reduces the ability to act rationally. Save important decisions or arguments for when you are feeling well, not zonked out.

Decreased alertness: This is particularly significant for shift-workers, or when you are performing monotonous tasks, but also affects your daily working life, certainly when you are trying to think or be creative. Since I've had insomnia, for example, my ability to write has been reduced by 50 per cent. These days I can't work for more than 3 hours at a stretch. Any longer and I find myself braindead and staring at a word that it takes me a minute to spell out, usually incorrectly. On a brighter note, studies show that you can function on 70 per cent of your normal sleep. Also, if you get about $5^{1}/_{2}$ hours' sleep, your performance will be no less than normal sleepers'. This is fine and dandy, but as insomniacs we know better than anyone else where our cut-off is in terms of performance: be aware of this, and make sure you adapt accordingly. You can always change the world later, or on really good days.

Driving: Despite what you think or however awake you may feel at the time, driving on little sleep is dangerous. The statistics on accidents caused by sleep-deprivation are horrendous. Get someone else to do the driving, or get a taxi/public transport.

Immune system: A lack of sleep leads to impaired immune system functioning. The result is fewer white cells to fight off invaders. This will not give you a heart attack, but will mean that your ability to ward off colds or viral infections or parasites is reduced, and you are more susceptible to being sick. If you are stressed it makes it worse, as the stress hormone cortisol has a powerful suppressing effect on the immune system as well. The immune system does not work in isolation, but talks to your brain and is intimately bound up with your circadian rhythms. The relationship is two-way – anything that upsets your immune system is likely to affect your sleep.

Your immune system recovers when your sleep does, but a struggling immune system is not a happy state, does not promote wellness, and is another good reason to do something about your insomnia *now.*

Memory: Sleep plays a large role in memory. Not surprisingly, then, your memory suffers when you persistently lack sleep. Learning new tasks is more difficult; you can't remember the words you want, and your mental clarity takes a nose-dive. This in turn leads to reduced self-confidence. Don't worry about this. It's temporary, and it's not your fault. Get on top of your insomnia, or rather the worry and anxiety it causes, and the clouds clear again.

Note: Memory impairment is a common side-effect of sleeping pills and anti-depressants, so if you are taking these to help you sleep, they may exacerbate the problem. This happened to me. You feel deranged, and it isn't nice.

Moods: There is no doubt that your outlook on life becomes more unpredictable, and generally shifts downwards. This is putting it diplomatically. Frustration, reduced motivation, feeling depressed or just feeling plain miserable happen quite a lot. What you must try your hardest to do is not to make this a way of life, as I did for a time. What you think, you become. *Don't* get used to being miserable at any cost. It's awful. And getting angry only makes matters worse. For more on this, and how not to succumb, see page 173.

David's story – get what you can

It is not only insomniacs who suffer the effects of sleep deprivation. David, 38, married with a family, works night-shift at the Royal Mail. Like countless thousands whose sleep-disruption is imposed on them due to their work, he lives with its debilitating effects. The cause is different, but the effects exactly the same.

> I've been working night-shifts in the sorting department at the Royal Mail for 6 years. I work a 4-day week, 6 p.m.–4 a.m., on a six-week rota, which means the days I am working also changes every 4 days. Apart from the fact that your sleep pattern is being constantly changed around, so is your diet. What to eat and when to eat it is an additional problem. On work days I will be in bed by 5 a.m. and sleep until 12–1 p.m. I fall asleep immediately but my sleep is very light – it's as if I've got one ear permanently tuned to whatever noise is around, and often wake up more tired than when I go to bed. I'm an owl by nature, so on non-work days I go to bed at 11 or 12 at night and will get up with the

family at 7.30–8 a.m., but will wake up frequently, so again constantly feel tired.

Working nights has had a huge effect on the quality of my sleep, and thus the way I am and the life I lead. It also has an effect on my family. I'm lucky I have a wife who is so supportive, but I see so many people who end up with relationship problems because of it. Speaking personally, I think the way employers disregard the sleep issue for anyone who works shifts is scandalous. It's the same with many of my colleagues. Most are on prescription drugs of some sort, or use alcohol to prop up the effects of just not getting regular sleep. I've had numerous ailments, am lethargic and am prone to depression. Not getting enough light (in winter I get about an hour) has a very real detrimental effect, also. I'm not an insomniac – I have the ability to sleep well, it's my job that sends it haywire. It's like living under a permanent fog. It's like you constantly have to work at being alive, or to want to do things. And you never feel well.

Progress: David has changed his job (he is now a gardener), and sleeps like a babe. For those who can't so easily manage to switch jobs, bright light therapy is commonly recommended to help shift-workers cope with their disrupted sleep (see page 194).

What's all the fuss about?

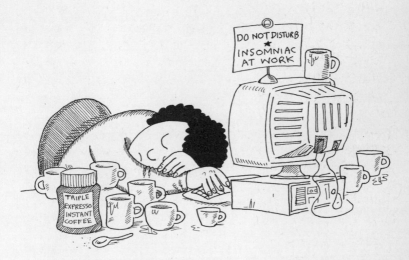

PART 2

Who are we?

How do I know
I'm an insomniac?

Millions of us don't sleep well, but have no idea whether we have insomnia or not, and therefore whether we should make an effort to resolve it, or struggle on hoping for a better night's sleep tonight – again.

What is insomnia?

Insomnia is not being able to sleep normally, by which I mean not being able to have an extended period of uninterrupted sleep that leaves you refreshed. It's finding sleep a struggle, instead of something that comes naturally.

Though insomniacs can spend whole nights awake, this does *not* mean no sleep. Insomnia is a state of being seriously sleepless to the extent that it impacts negatively on your waking life; for many of us, not sleeping well dominates our lives. Whether you experience insomnia most of the time or only intermittently, it feels the same and sets off the same vicious circle.

Insomnia is also a subjective state. As Dr Dilys Davies in *Insomnia, Your Questions Answered* puts it, you are the best judge of whether or not you are an insomniac. Don't let anyone else tell you otherwise.

It's important to realize from the outset, too, that though countless books have been written on the subject, despite the impression given insomnia can't be neatly pigeon-holed. Its causes and the way it expresses itself are too varied to bear absolute generalization.

That said, working out whether you are 'officially' an insomniac is easy. In a nutshell, if you can't fall asleep or stay asleep, can't get back to sleep, and feel deprived of the benefits of sleep, you're an insomniac.

The three prime symptoms of insomnia recognized by sleep scientists are:

1. Difficulty getting off to sleep (sleep-onset insomnia): Normal sleepers take anywhere from 1–20 minutes to fall asleep. Insomniacs habitually take longer: 30 minutes and upwards, the average time being about $1^1/4$ hours. Moreover, we can find it extremely difficult to get to sleep irrespective of how tired we are, or how little sleep we may have had the previous night(s). If your insomnia is confined to not being able to fall asleep, the cause (or one of them) is likely to be that your body clock is running too late. See pages 15 and 194.

2. Persistent waking up (sleep-maintenance insomnia): During the course of normal sleep, everyone wakes up momentarily – but we are not aware of this, so sleep seems unbroken. It's quite natural, too, to wake up if you're too hot or too cold, need to visit the bathroom, there's a dog barking, you've got a plane to catch, an important exam the next morning, etc. For an insomniac, however, waking up, and the inevitable tossing and turning and frustration because we can't get back to sleep, is the norm. For some of us, myself included, we can either be awake for hours, or we can wake so often that sleep seems like an extended period of short naps and a perpetual state of being half-awake and never quite asleep.

Sleep scientists reckon that being awake for 30 minutes or more during the night is enough to qualify for sleep-maintenance insomnia; again, the average is about $1^1/4$ hours.

3. Early morning waking: Waking up early is not a symptom of insomnia. Millions of larks, and people who have a good night's sleep, do so daily. Millions of people, too, choose to get up early – and generally compensate by going to bed earlier than most of us. Waking early and not being able to go back to sleep as the norm, however, after sleep-deprived nights, and persistently waking up earlier than you feel you need, are symptoms of insomnia. If your insomnia is confined to persistently waking up earlier, two common

z z z z

causes are depression or a body clock that is running too early. For more on this, see pages 15 and 194.

If you experience any, all or any combination of the three symptoms above, you have insomnia. In the US, to 'qualify' as an insomniac you must typically take at least 30 minutes to fall asleep, sleep fewer than six hours and/or wake up frequently, though increasingly sleep doctors rely more on the subjective diagnosis of the patient.

If the symptoms are temporary – lasting less than a month, due to whatever cause – don't be unduly concerned, though do make an effort to do the simple things outlined in Part 3 to help you sleep better and restore your natural sleep patterns sooner. If your symptoms persist for more than a month, you qualify, medically speaking, as a chronic insomniac and you *must* do something about it.

The WORRY factor

The symptoms above are physical, measurable symptoms, and when you complete a sleep diary these are the things to note down. However, there is a fourth, equally important symptom that sets many ordinary insomniacs and people who suffer from sleep deprivation apart from the rest: WORRY.

There are many people who, for whatever reason, do not sleep well, but who don't worry about it. Conversely, many others I've spoken to regularly manage to sleep five hours and more – and worry like mad. It is those of us who worry persistently, and for whom sleep becomes a Big Issue that impacts on our lives negatively – and sometimes disastrously – that qualify as insomniacs. Sleep specialists confirm that many people who 'whinge' about insomnia actually get as much sleep as people who don't feel they've got insomnia, or who do not feel deprived of sleep. This is true – and has been recorded umpteen times in sleep laboratories – but misses the point. If you feel that sleep is a real problem for you, in this book you've got insomnia. For more on what it feels like, see page 57.

z z z z

Insomnia: a symptom, not a disease

A persistent theme throughout the book, but one worth repeating and reminding ourselves about because it holds the ultimate key to long-term relief, is that insomnia is neither a disease nor an illness but a collection of symptoms (orthodox view) or state of imbalance (holistic view). Remedies that tackle only the symptoms are usually helpful, but don't take on the underlying cause. As holistic practitioners often remind me, it's a question of removing the 'dis-ease' from our disease.

Where I take issue, however, is that I believe it is actually useful to think of insomnia as an illness. It's easier to deal with in your head, and for those you live with, too. In my own case, it was when I and my husband finally acknowledged that I was ill, in the sense of being on the edge and permanently fragile, that made all the difference with coping with my insomnia. It also gave me permission to be ill, if you see what I mean, instead of berating myself because I couldn't sleep and desperately trying (and failing) to be normal. Whether it's short or long term, whatever the cause, and whether it's self-induced or not, being sleep-deprived *is* a serious issue; if it helps to see it as an illness (after all, we all get ill, and all recover), so be it.

For more on the symptoms of insomnia, see page 43.

For more on insomnia as imbalance, see page 30.

Insomnia is unique

Though we all talk about the same sort of symptoms and experience the same sort of problems, everyone's insomnia is different and unique to us. By the same token, the solution will be unique to you. Grasp this and you're well on the way to your first step to resolving it.

Insomnia doesn't happen all the time

Just as it is a myth that insomniacs never sleep at all, many long-term insomniacs have periods when their sleep is reasonable; this is one reason why intermittent insomniacs like Maria (page 36) put up with it, even though it rules their lives. Those of us who suffer poor-to-awful sleep as a matter of course also find that insomnia can wax and wane, and that the pattern of our sleeplessness can change.

Learned insomnia

A bitter pill to swallow, but many of the problems associated with chronic insomnia are self-inflicted – in the sense that we have literally learned not to sleep. This is known as *psychophysiological insomnia*. I was (am) a textbook case. The good news is, something you have learned can be unlearned. This is the basis of the behavioural methods to cure insomnia. Indeed, for long-term progress, whichever 'cure' you find, you are going to have to change your mindset from negative 'can't' to positive 'can' in some way. For how, see page 176.

Self-imposed sleep-deprivation vs insomnia

Working shifts, jet-lag, sitting exams, having a baby or finding yourself in a holiday cottage next to a railway line can all cause severe sleep problems. The critical difference, however, between this kind of imposed sleep-deprivation and insomnia is that there is tangible relief ahead: like David (page 45), you still have the ability to sleep when circumstances allow it, or the situation changes. Insomniacs don't have that luxury, and have to work much harder to re-establish what everyone else takes for granted – a God-given ability to sleep.

Core characteristics of insomnia

It is easy to get confused when reading up on sleep and insomnia. On one hand, sleep science seems fairly straightforward to understand; on the other, every sleep expert has his or her own spin. In reality, for ordinary insomniacs whose insomnia can't be pinpointed as a sleep disorder or obvious medical condition, it's much simpler. The core characteristics of insomnia can be boiled down to four key factors:

1. Worry/stress/anxiety is constant. The only difference is how high or low the volume.

2. A fragile nature: *anything, absolutely anything,* disrupts our sleep.
3. Unpredictability: insomnia has a mind of its own and comes and goes whenever it likes, often out of the blue.
4. Disturbed sleep/short sleep: irrespective of when we get to sleep or when we wake up, we either get an awful lot of disturbed sleep, get only short amounts of unbroken sleep, or both.

Types of insomnia

Sleep scientists distinguish three basic types – though don't worry if your insomnia doesn't exactly fit one of them.

1. *Transient insomnia*: This lasts for a few nights and is due to changes in your normal sleep schedule such as jet-lag, illness, over-excitement, etc. This accounts for about 75 per cent of all insomnia cases.
2. *Short-term insomnia*: This lasts for three to four weeks and is generally due to more prolonged periods of stress such as bereavement, financial troubles, relationship problems, etc. If not addressed, it may (and usually does) escalate into full-blown chronic insomnia.
3. *Chronic insomnia*: This is long-term insomnia, insomnia that lasts for a month or more. It can be caused by any number of factors, including those that are not evident at the time, or just bad sleep habits. It can last for a few months or several years, though this is rarer. As mentioned above, it can occur every night, most nights or intermittently – but never goes away!

Idiopathic insomnia

A few people develop insomnia during childhood, and have a life-long inability to get adequate sleep. Adam (page 74) is one, as is Wendy (see page 64). The cause is unknown but presumed to be an abnormality in the sleep-wake system mechanism of the brain.

Sleep-state misperception

Some unfortunate insomniacs believe and experience insomnia and live with its debilitating effects, yet when tested in a sleep laboratory show completely normal sleep patterns. The only way of finding this out is to be tested. Again, the cause is unknown, but it is presumed that these people have a higher brain activity which makes them think they are awake, even though they are asleep.

Sleep-disorder insomniacs

Insomnia is a feature of many recognized sleep disorders. Many insomniacs are unaware of this. Sleep-disorder centres and clinics are the only places where you can find out whether this applies to you.

Which sounds like you?

The book *Beating Insomnia* spins the wheel slightly differently, and categorizes the kind of insomniac you are in a more qualitative way – helpful when trying to separate the scientific gobbledegook from what is driving your insomnia at an emotional level. Drugs, depression, alcoholism and circadian rhythm imbalance are included in this list, as well as the following:

Anxiety insomnia	Where anxiety rules, manifested by general anxiety, tension and feeling on edge, and by physical symptoms such as butterflies in the stomach, frequent diarrhoea, dry mouth, etc.
Tension insomnia	Where stress and tension rule, manifested in an inability to relax, muscle ache, headaches, finding it hard to let go.
Sleep-centred insomnia	Obsession with not sleeping well/enough, and believing that you can't cope, can't concentrate, feel unwell, look awful, etc. if you don't get enough sleep.

| Stimulus-control insomnia | Being awake, watching TV in bed; falling asleep somewhere other than your bed (e.g. the living room) or sleeping better in a bed which isn't yours. |
| Worry-centred insomnia | Worrying about not being to sleep, being unable to unwind, worrying about the day, the next day, the day after ... |

The other dimensions of sleep

Spiritual and vibrational (energy) medicine perspectives shed their own light on not being able to sleep. Briefly, sleep is thought to be necessary because our nervous system and minds are troubled and stressed; a calm mind, which is well trained and has a positive attitude, needs less sleep or no sleep. Indeed, for advanced meditators it is possible to use sleep as a means of attaining a degree of enlightenment called 'the clear state'.

For those of us who can't sleep, the mind is so distracted and agitated that it is unable to relax. It's like having a polluted mind: for whatever reason, we collect, or have collected, more than our share of the negative debris of everyday life. (Don't forget, either, that there's a two-way interchange between body and mind: physical and emotional information stored at the molecular level in the body also impacts profoundly on sleep.) As one meditation teacher explains, the mind is the conveyor of consciousness, and what we make of the world depends on which level of consciousness we abide in. Another interpretation offered to me was that not being able to sleep was like having an inflamed central nervous system, which means the mind gets no relief and that, in some way and at some level, we don't want or are unable to come to terms with our Being. So we stay awake or have nightmares instead.

Vibrational energy medicine sees human beings as dynamic multi-dimensional, energetic beings. Our physical bodies are but one realm or dimension we occupy; the others – namely the

z Z z z

etheric, astral, mental, causal, Buddhic and atmic, which collectively make up the auric field – are our higher vibrational energy fields or spiritual planes that are connected to the vibrational universe from whence we came and where we eternally belong. It's believed, for example, that while we are sleeping and dreaming, our spirit leaves us and occupies the astral plane; indeed, out-of-body 'dreams' are a recognized phenomena.

Deep sleep is also the state of nothingness (what, as insomniacs, we yearn for most). When we can't sleep, our Spirit remains stuck in our physical and etheric bodies. This prevents our minds from acquiring 'death' – that is, that state of nothingness which regenerates us. To put it another way, not sleeping means the computer (conscious mind) is always on-line, denying us the opportunity to connect with our higher selves via dreams and our subconscious. The left brain (logic centre) wins, and the right brain (our creative side) loses out.

As touched on elsewhere, the view of sleep as a death state is recognized by both Western and Eastern philosophies. It's the state where, generally at least, we have no control. The fear of this – which is primeval – keeps some of us awake.

A sobering thought, but we may also choose not to sleep as an avoidance tactic. As Hiliary Luxton, a communications therapist, puts it, 'Perhaps we are removing the one thing we need to stay balanced and healthy – sleep and dreaming – because it just hurts too much right now to face it all.' If it's a soul journey, then perhaps our soul is creating conditions that are so unbearable that eventually we will be forced to change – or, in soul-speak, evolve. As far as our soul is concerned, this change is always for our good.

Insomnia's incestuous nature

Insomnia is incestuous by nature. The symptoms of everyday insomnia thrive on each other and are inextricably bound up with each other. You begin by not sleeping well for a few nights; this

z z z z

makes you anxious, which exacerbates your inability to sleep. A few nights more and your body clock is all over the place, reducing your ability to sleep further. You, meanwhile, get more tired, more anxious and more prone to staying in bed to see if you can catch up on sleep. You may become too tired to eat well, or start drinking more coffee during the day to keep you awake, and more alcohol at night to put you to sleep. The cumulative effect of all of this affects what's happening bio-chemically. Stress hormones, notably adrenaline and cortisol, kick in and do their best to keep you on red alert. You produce less serotonin and melatonin, which means you don't have the right amount of bio-chemical tackle, as it were, to sleep. And so it goes on … and on. This is why you need to find the keys that will help you break the cycle; and why the set of keys that will unlock your insomnia will be specific to you.

How severe is my insomnia?

The simplest way to work this out is to keep a sleep diary for one to two weeks. There are three good reasons for this:

1. It will change what you think and feel into fact. Once you find a pattern for your insomnia, you will be able to begin to assess your insomnia in a tangible, pragmatic way. This gives you the first valuable clues to how you can manage your sleep habits to give you better sleep.
2. Sleep specialists love them, and will ask you to do one before you see them.
3. General practitioners are impressed and will take your plea for help more seriously if they know you are serious about it, too.

Sleep diaries

Most books on insomnia will include a sample sleep diary. Mine is on page 287. Please remember that the pattern of your disturbed sleep pattern can change – mine has gone through at least two major shifts in the last three years, so though keeping a sleep diary will give

zZzᶻ

you a revealing and much more accurate snapshot of your insomnia now, it isn't necessarily a permanent blueprint.

Are there any downsides to keeping a sleep diary? Yes. It does mean actively engaging with how bad or good your sleep is, which can be unbalancing, at least temporarily. I know some insomniacs who flatly refuse to do one, simply because they don't want to be reminded about last night's sleep. I myself have been at the stage where I couldn't face continuing to do one, albeit under professional guidance, for that same reason. But, this apart, if you want to take control over your sleeplessness, a sleep diary really is a very good idea.

Insomniac's sleep

The word that constantly comes to mind that best describes an insomniac's sleep is 'fragile'. An insomniac's sleep is a delicate, elusive prize that we struggle to capture and which can be broken with a feather. The slightest noise, emotional upset or change to our routine and it all goes pear-shaped again. Often it goes pear-shaped for no reason, which is doubly frustrating and sends panic messages round your system.

Insomniacs sleep differently from normal sleepers. It's well documented, for example, that we spend more time in light sleep. Studies show that insomniacs have faster brain patterns than normal sleepers, faster heart rates and more muscle tension through the night; predictably, we also have higher levels of stress hormones, which is probably why our hearts are beating faster. Our body temperature takes longer to drop in the evening, and doesn't drop as much as that of normal sleepers. Generally our body temperature doesn't fluctuate as much as other people's (though part of the reason for this is that we go round in a daze and are often too tired to exercise). Apparently, our sleep-wake system doesn't function properly, either. Our sleep system is either too weak, or our wake system is too strong. We spend more time in Stage 1 and 2 sleep, and often go without as much REM sleep as we need. Do you need or want to know any more?

z z z z

Lady of the night

Talk to insomniacs and we all have our own graphic descriptions of what insomnia is. This is Geraldene's:

> Insomnia is a coquettish, fickle, precocious lady of the night. A courtesan who refuses to be courted. You do everything to placate her, please her, woo her, pander to her every whim – and still she will not yield, and allow you to partake of her charms. There are times when I am at a loss as to what to do, and can't for the life of me understand. 'Why me? Why am I afflicted this way, and why is she always so elusive or difficult? After all, it's only a bit of decent sleep I want!'

How many hours of sleep?

As a rough rule of thumb, sleep specialists reckon if you spend around 85 per cent of your time in bed asleep, you are getting the required amount of sleep for you; if you frequently spend less time than this asleep, you are probably suffering from chronic insomnia.

However, don't take this too literally. Some of us just like being in bed. Or like lying in. Sometimes you just have to use your common sense, and just as I believe it is really important to a find out whether you are an insomniac, it's equally important *not* to convince yourself you are one if you aren't. Being sleep-deprived, for example, doesn't necessarily make you an insomniac. You may simply be a short sleeper, or need to acknowledge that as time ticks by your sleep can expect to get lighter and more fragmented. If this is the case, you need to make some adjustments to your lifestyle, and your mental outlook, to ensure you get the best sleep you can, and are content with that; what you don't need is to worry yourself to death about the fact that your best friend or partner gets more sleep than you do.

What kind of insomniac am I?

The medical definitions outlined at the beginning of this chapter are fine for doctors, and have their place, but start talking to ordinary insomniacs or people worried about their lack of decent kip and it quickly becomes apparent that, in real life, we fall into different sorts of groups. This is how I see 'normal' insomniacs – that is, those of us who become insomniacs for no obvious reason. If this definition works for you, use it to help you work out your strategy for tackling your sleep problem. If it doesn't, don't worry.

Temporary insomniacs
Have short-term insomnia due to an unforseen/unexpected external event. This is the easiest type of insomnia to deal with and overcome.

Straightforward insomniacs
May have had insomnia for some time, but their insomnia is due to a simple or relatively simple cause – physical, mental or emotional. The cause may have started in childhood, but can be pinpointed. Again, though it takes more effort, and different solutions will need to be tried, it can be cured. It will need more than a stab in the dark, however. Some insomniacs I have talked to in this group, such as Helen (page 141), lack the motivation to find a solution because they have learned to live with their insomnia. Wanting to make the effort can be the first important step for them.

Complex insomniacs
The complicated, complex, muddled-up sort whose insomnia is an infernal network of causes, some easy to spot, some unknown or buried deep in our subconscious or medical history. Unless you're very lucky, treatment for this type needs to be thorough and systematic, may be long term, and will probably require drastic options such as sleep-restriction therapy or regression hynotherapy. This type of insomnia subdivides into people with:

Chronic insomnia - or - **Wake-up call insomnia**	The insomnia that most people with long-term insomnia identify with The bottom (or top) of the pile (depending on how you view it). This is the group I put myself in. Insomnia is a tool that our body/mind/spirit keeps us awake with because the time has come to face up to ourselves and our lives.

Insomniacs in every group will probably have some learned insomnia, and the usual rat-bag of symptoms. I also figure that the more complicated your insomnia, the more effort you will have to put in to find the remedies and cures that will turn the corner for you, and the more willpower to help your SELF you will need.

If all this sounds like the dis-ease is easier to cope with than the cure, don't believe it for a second. *Better sleep changes everything.* The journey to achieving this may not be pleasant, but will enrich you and lead you places you never thought you'd go. Though it sounds ridiculous, one day you may even, like me, look back and be grateful for your insomnia.

Real-life insomniacs

To prove the point that neither insomnia nor insomniacs can be neatly pigeonholed, two typically atypical stories:

Wendy's story – the perverse insomniac

Wendy, 37, works in publishing and is a life-long insomniac.

My mother and sister are both insomniacs. Mine developed when I was a child and I used to write 'worry lists' to take my mind off things when I went to bed. By the time I was 14, I was having nights without sleep. My insomnia, however, has always been intermittent. I sleep normally for a few weeks, then it hits me. The pattern is always the same: a night with no sleep which leaves me, perversely, feeling very light-headed, lively and 'high' for the next 24 hours – like the feeling you get when you've had a good all-night-out on the town. Another night with no sleep and a couple more nights with minimal sleep follow, with the usual drastic side-effects. By the fifth night my body says 'enough', the madness stops and I return to normal sleep.

It dominates my life, and I'm just as obsessive as most insomniacs, but though I dabble, I've never really seriously tried to do anything about it. I just manage it in my own idiosyncratic way. I think it's because I'm a 'blocker-outer' rather than an 'analyser' and have an almost superstitious fear of talking about it in case it makes me even more neurotic.

Progress: Wendy has now met the love of her life, who happens to be a snorer. From the outset, they took the decision to have separate bedrooms. They are now engaged and Wendy is sleeping much better. Congratulations all round.

Will's story – the reformed insomniac

Will, 52, works in insurance. His story is typical – but also shows there is a way through.

I was a happy child who slept well. Then something happened. I think it was probably the stress caused by frequent rows between my parents and starting secondary school. Anyway, my sleep became very erratic and I began having headaches, which developed into severe migraines. By the time I was adult and working, the fear of having 'a bad head', which I would have every couple of weeks, got worse and became a constant preoccupation, especially if I had an important meeting the following day. My sleeping pattern remained like this from adolescence until two years ago: I'd manage a couple of hours when I went to bed, wake up around 1-ish, and begin the nightly vigil of trying and mostly failing to get back to sleep. I would wake just before daylight, toss and turn a bit longer and then get up feeling heavy, lethargic and knackered. I never tried to do anything about it, accepting it as my lot. At weekends I would nap for a few minutes in the afternoon, which helped.

My sister suggested I see her chiropracter. He miraculously fixed my migraines. That led me to Network Spinal Care (a specialized chiropractic technique which involves gentle adjustments and developing deep breath), and then to the well-known dowser and healer Jack Temple.

Today, I'm a new man. My sleep has improved, not drastically, but I no longer worry about it. Curing my migranes took away the lifelong fear of what not sleeping well meant to me. I've learned I only need four to five hours' sleep, that going to bed early is right for me and that adopting a positive attitude – by being more relaxed about my sleep – takes away most of the anxiety that has been my life. I know I'm a very light sleeper, and need to take care of that. I know that what I eat affects my sleep – as does which way my bed is facing – and am generally just much more mindful these days and have a better ability to tune in to myself. Technically I'm still an insomniac – I wake up early and rarely get more than three hours' unbroken sleep – but am no longer knackered. Most days now I wake up feeling energized, and when my sleep does get seriously disturbed, I feel I'm in a much better position to help myself.

Progress: When I last checked, Will was normally getting a good four hours' straight sleep and getting off to sleep within 10 minutes – with very little anxiety at all.

z z z z

Who we are and how insomnia affects our lives

Insomniacs come in all shapes and sizes and from all walks of life. Statistically the only two groups who are more prone to insomnia are middle-aged women and the elderly. On the whole, too, we're a pretty nice, normal bunch who happen to have got ourselves into a sleepless mess and who have to cope with the consequences. We are not necessarily neurotic, maladapted, sad people who find life difficult or stressful (though sleeplessness itself can have this effect). In fact, about a third of the population are programmed to be poor sleepers should life go temporarily pear-shaped, and it's estimated that, at any given time, up to 15 per cent or more of the population – some estimates put it as high as 25 per cent – experience insomnia; 4 million of us in the UK are complaining of chronic insomnia right now.

Though we're all very different, there's no doubt we have a lot of behavioural traits in common. For example, have you ever met anyone who is proud to be an insomniac? On the contrary, we all feel bad, mad or boring about it, and most of us feel guilty in some way – we see it as sort of letting the side down. As a result, many of us find talking to normal sleepers generally embarrassing: this is because we either feel bad for talking about it, or they feel bad because they are powerless to help. Put two or more insomniacs together and, hey presto, the floodgates open. All of a sudden we can bore each other stupid over how much sleep we haven't had, go into endless detail about last night's lack of sleep, how we are feeling (usually crap), how tired we are, our current theories of why we

z z z z

can't sleep this week but could last week, the latest miracle cure, and so on.

We are all acutely aware, too, that unless our insomnia is caused by, for example, a physical sleep disorder, medical problem or one of life's regular hiccups, we alone are responsible: we do it to ourselves.

So, sorry, but no excuses that this section makes for pretty dismal reading: not sleeping *is* pretty dismal. But there is one bright note. On good days, insomniacs really shine. It's like being let out of prison: your appreciation of life, however ordinary and humdrum, is doubled. The world tastes sweet and full of promise again, and you relish every single minute. Sounds daft, but I have literally experienced bliss on occasion.

How common is insomnia?

Insomnia is more common than you think. It is reckoned to be the most common complaint after headaches. Almost all (95 per cent) people will experience the odd bout of insomnia at some time in their lives. Most people who have insomnia don't seek medical help. Insomnia is also on the increase. This is no comfort for an insomniac, but at least we know we are not alone, and are much more normal after all.

The struggle

Sleep scientists comment that insomniac patients often describe getting enough sleep as the greatest struggle in their lives. It's true. It can seem like an insurmountable, slippery mountain that you are forced to climb every day. Hang in there.

Being tired

The tiredness that insomniacs experience is not like the tiredness that most of us feel after a bad night's sleep or after intense physical activity, or even the general tiredness that seems a common factor of modern life. Indeed, although insomnia's a trial, often you can cope physically – I know insomniacs who cycle to work and, like me, wouldn't miss their salsa class for anything, however tired they may be. An insomniac's tiredness is a multi-dimensional phenomenon that permeates every fibre of your being, eats into your soul and, drip by drip, depletes your vitality and robs you of the Real You. There is the constant weariness associated with putting a brave face on it, being normal and getting on with your life feeling permanently zapped and emotionally frazzled yet powerless to do anything about it. It knaws away at your self-confidence and self-esteem, and anxiety and often depression hover around like waiting jackals. The fact that it's written all over your face – and you're fed up of looking at that shagged-out, ashen-faced creature – doesn't help.

Mentally, too, this kind of tiredness has a quality all its own. One of the worst aspects of insomnia tiredness, for example, is its ability to consume you completely. So much so that it becomes the focus of your consciousness to the exclusion of the external world around you. In short, it dominates your thoughts as well as your actions. Another big difference between insomniacs and other people is that we get so little rest from ourselves. We live with ourselves and our thoughts night and day. Indeed, for an insomniac, an important function of sleep that is denied to us, which most people take for granted, is having that break from our brains. Unlike everyone else, mentally speaking we have nowhere to run to in the middle of the night. It's what people who meditate call the 'chatter' of the mind. It is as debilitating as lack of sleep itself, and normal sleepers have no idea what a precious prize being relieved of yourself can be.

The tiredness varies from day to day, and you become so attuned to it that you can literally measure what kind of day you can expect as soon as you wake up – and make adjustments accordingly, whether this means 'closing down' for the day, putting off that important meeting, going to the supermarket or, yet again, cancelling that evening out. If the night yields below the minimum number of hours you need to function, bleary and very sore eyes, or nausea and loss of appetite, for example, for some of us can become the norm, and even if we have the energy to cook, we can't find the energy to eat.

The two yous

Apart from the tiredness, or probably because of it, persistent insomnia often changes your personality and how you view yourself:

The Real You is the person you are after a reasonable night's sleep. This is the You you know and understand reasonably well, that your family and friends love, and that your colleagues are familiar with. The Other You is an emotionally fraught, grey being who can't think straight, who doesn't engage with the world, who is anxious, apathetic, lethargic and nervy. Someone who is permanently enveloped in a cloak of negativity, and for whom the self-inflicted doubts and worries that inevitably arise can seem very real. Coping with this Other You can be as difficult as insomnia itself, and for some causes far more concern than lack of sleep. No one describes this better than Nick (below).

Ring any bells? If so, it's important for all concerned, especially you, to recognize these personality changes and understand that they are genuinely *not* really you, any more than the fog of negativity surrounding you is really real. It is also the quickest and easiest route I have found to preserving your sanity.

Nick's story – on being an insomniac

Nick's insomnia was caused by a severe illness in his early twenties, compounded by two years' working nights. Now in his early forties, his insomnia, which he understands and manages well, has persisted for 20 years. Few people understand its effects better.

After a bad night it's important to me to 'come out' and say 'I'm an insomniac, so please make allowances today,' so normal people won't judge me by the person they see who is functioning well under par. There is a sense of social isolation and paranoia – I worry that people think I'm weird in some way, a bit anti-social, a bit of a drag, not good company, and that I'm slow and can't think as clearly as I should. There is also the

z z z z

frustration of being robbed not only of your potential but the day's potential: that 'another-day-lost' sinking feeling which becomes part of daily life. The tiredness is all-pervading and I can tell by how knackered I look in the morning what kind of day it will be. On a really bad day I feel like the living dead, dejected and dis-empowered. I draw in and connect only with my own tired, internal world. During the day at work I put on a mask – it's important to remain positive in your job, but inevitably, though I try, the irritability, impatience, moodiness and general emotional spikiness which accompanies insomnia is more difficult to control at home.

As an insomniac you can get by on 80 per cent of your faculties; it's the 20 per cent you don't have that makes the real difference I find, particularly at work, and if possible I'll put off the more intellectually demanding tasks until I've got a better night's sleep.

Otherwise, these days I remain positive – I'm quite cool about my insomnia; it doesn't control my life completely. I remind myself constantly that though my insomnia poses limitations on what I can and can't do, I'm never less as a person and I always do have that potential to be the person I want and live life to the full. Two nights' good sleep turns things around instantly. The clouds part, doubts melt away, the world changes from grey to full colour again – and I become the real, rested me: I feel bright, energetic, happy, am more entertaining, see and feel more, am in touch with the world again, feel my own potency and vitality and am keen to get out and savour every precious second of the day.

Being obsessional

Though we hide it pretty well in public, and there are many exceptions (if you are one, count your blessings), as anyone who lives with an insomniac will tell you, we can be (and usually are) completely obsessional about our lack of sleep. This takes many forms, from the rituals that surround bedtime to what you will or won't eat, will or won't do, and to how we plan life generally. Talking incessantly about how you do and don't sleep when you get the chance is just the tip of the obsessional iceberg – friends and family beware. For what's it like, see Richard's story (page 81).

z z z z

As insomniacs understand well, sleep is not just a physiological response. Mind (and spirit) play major roles. Maggie Peters, who has over 20 years' experience in transpersonal psychotherapy, counselling and dream therapy, and author of *Dreamwork – Using Your Dreams as the Way to Self-discovery and Personal Development*, explains who we are this way:

> As a psychotherapist I have come to understand that those suffering from insomnia, if they can be generalized at all, are people who live at a high level of arousal. Unconsciously they seem to feel they have to maintain hyper-vigilance to keep themselves safe within their environment and relationships. This suggests that at some time, often but not exclusively in early childhood, their support system has severely failed them and they have felt that they had to totally support themselves. This belief, if left unchallenged, will dominate their responses to life. Adaptive behaviour results.
>
> Insomnia may not kick in until later in life when a similar loss of support may evoke the feelings and deep anxiety which have been repressed by good coping mechanisms. Repeat incidences of failure of support systems, coupled with attempts to subdue or deny the deep feeling responses they evoke, will eventually lead to a stress overload. The system is experiencing more than it is able or allowed to process, which leads to an intolerable level of chronic stress that can result in insomnia, illness, serious accidents and breakdown.

Sense and non-sense

One of the most frustrating aspects of insomnia is that there is often no rhyme nor reason to the pattern of our sleeping/not-sleeping. It can be totally unpredictable. Your life can be calm, you can be calm – and yet inexplicably you can have a run of really bad sleep. Don't expect insomnia to make sense. And as we can't make sense of it, it's unfair to expect anyone else to make sense of it, either.

Self-pity

We do this too, though mainly in the middle of night and in private.

Life

Is on hold quite a lot of the time. You tend to do the minimum, and are constantly re-evaluating what you can/can't and should/shouldn't do. Sad to say, but insomnia makes you a more cautious, less outgoing, fun person than you used to be. We also view making plans differently. On the whole we try and not make them unless absolutely necessary, especially social engagements. This is because you can never be sure just how you are going to feel. Really bad insomnia means survival tactics: you put off everything except absolutely essential tasks.

Daily life inevitably revolves around how much sleep we have or haven't had the night before, and therefore how well we are likely to cope during the day. If you are working, your preoccupation is about how well you can do your job that day, how impaired your performance is, and how much your colleagues will notice. If you have children, there's the pressure to be bright, cheerful and caring, even though it is you who craves the being looked after. If you're at home like me, though you can hate yourself for it, it's much easier to give into the tiredness – isn't it amazing how much hard work it is to take the rubbish to the dustbin?

Relationships

One of the most stressful aspects of coping with insomnia is relationships: at work, home and within your social circle. Feeling that you are not performing as well as you can causes a great deal of anxiety. Regrettably we don't have a culture that makes allowances for lack of sleep, so at work insomniacs develop various coping devices. Alas, drinking strong coffee is a common one; putting off important meetings or writing that important report are others. Often we just simply hide it and put on a public face of normality. Finding other insomniacs is a big

z z z z

help. I know of one threesome who operate their own chatline and send each other emails with snippets of info/ advice, etc.

Adam's story – an insomniac at work

Adam is another life-long insomniac, who manages his insomnia this way.

> I'll always make sure my morning routine is taken very slowly if I've been sleeping badly, and especially if I haven't slept at all. If I'm already awake but still in bed, then I open the window as wide as I can to get some air flowing through the lungs. A long hot shower is a must, as is a big breakfast (plus banana if required!).
>
> When tired, I'll try and get regular breaks from the desk – and I'll always try and get a full hour's lunch if possible. The late afternoons tend to be the trickiest part of the day, so at this point I'll be drinking shed loads of water and popping outside for five minutes of fresh air and maybe a quick walk to the newsagent's. As I don't drink tea or coffee, my weakness at such points is a can of cola.
>
> After a few days without sleep the world at large does tend to take on an almost unreal appearance, as if my senses are delaying everything, so I just take things carefully and ensure this doesn't affect work quality. The only specific problem is eye-ache from staring at a computer screen with already-tired eyes, so again if the day can be 'mixed up' a little – with regular breaks doing other types of work – then I'll do that.

Friends

Though you can hide insomnia from your work colleagues and in the company of people you don't know well, it is impossible to do so with close friends. And as in any life crisis, it is your close friends who usually turn up trumps: they listen to you endlessly, offer constant support, don't mind your rituals or the fact that you regularly go AWOL, and even drive you around when necessary (thank you, Catey). The great thing about close friends is that they don't live with you. That makes the relationship stress-free – and makes a couple of good friends one of the best medicines you can hope for.

Holidays

Can become a double whammy. As I know from personal experience, for an insomniac, a holiday can quickly become an ordeal rather than a pleasure, and a source of extra pressure rather than a release. You're too tired to enjoy yourself, you are not fun to be with, and there's the jet-lag, strange bed, odd mealtimes, too much booze, high temperature, etc. to cope with as well. The real holiday would be to let the rest of the family go off and leave you at home. Or going with friends who graciously understand your peccadillos and foibles. At the very least, organize things so you can have a separate bedroom if you need it.

And so to bed ...

An insomniac's bedroom is a cross between a shrine to peace and an obstacle course. It is here that the obsessional nature of an insomniac finds its ultimate expression. What we want is absolute dark, absolute quiet, no interruptions whatsoever, and an absolute right to conduct our nightly ritual, whatever that may be, which has been carefully and idiosyncratically designed to lull us into sleep. To illustrate the point, I once shared a room with a girlfriend on a weekend away. She watched in disbelief as I first got out all my various bottles and potions (lavender and sandlewood essential oils, Bach Flower remedies, etc.). Next came the sleeping tablet carefully placed on the bedside table (just in case), along with my nice blue crystal. My personal stereo containing stress and insomnia tapes was rigged up, and my 'pillow talk' headphone positioned in place under my pillow. The sound was checked, ready to go. The hotel room clock was then turned away so I couldn't see it: if it ticked, it would have had to be wrapped in a spare blanket or jumper. A large glass of water was placed near my bed, with the bottle close by in case I needed extra. The main light was immediately switched off. On my pillow, I placed an eye patch (this was for the dawn shift). I then got into bed, dabbed lavender on my wrists and soles of my feet, draped my piece of Thai silk doused with fresh sandlewood over my face, and spent two minutes cradling the back of my neck in my magic pillow. If I'd been at home, a glass of hot organic milk and grated nutmeg would be *de rigeur.* This, or something similar, is normal for me. These days, a nightly bath (see page 147), candles and overnight tapes/CDs are must-have essentials, too. It's called clutching at straws, and sorry, but we honestly can't help it.

What we think of our beds

There is much talk in books on insomnia or how to sleep well about having a positive approach to your bed, and seeing bed as a haven of comfort, pregnant with sleep and relaxing thoughts. Though some insomniacs do fear their beds, this is not always the case. Many of us, myself included, love our beds, and it's just as much our comfort zone as it is for normal sleepers. It's being awake that's the problem, not being in bed. Paradoxically, bed can seem its nicest in the morning when you have to get up: you're exhausted, it's too late for sleep and your bed seems a much better place than the reality you will face when you get up.

Lights

Are anathema to us. This includes the main light in the bedroom, landing or anywhere else that could possibly come into our view. If we get up, whereas most people would put on a light to find their way to the loo or wherever, we stumble around in the dark. We get very good at doing this. We know it doesn't make sense, but the fear that a light, however dim, can wake us up further is all we need to remain steadfast moles. This is also partly why some insomniacs, including myself, find advice about getting up in the middle of night and doing some light task difficult to swallow.

How we view sleep

The observation that we regularly underestimate how much sleep we actually manage to bag is true. Where sleep is concerned, our glasses

z z z z

are permanently half-empty and you will rarely hear an insomniac say, 'I had a good night's sleep last night.' Unless we hit the magic jackpot – namely around eight hours' of uninterrupted sleep – even if we do get a decent night's sleep we tend to qualify it as 'good for me', or 'good by my standards'. This can be infuriating for family and friends, who are doing their best to bolster you up. We don't do this to get extra sympathy, however. It's simply that where sleep is concerned, we quickly learn to take one day at a time and never be too optimistic. In this sense it's like being a reformed alcoholic. It's a defence mechanism, first to remind you to be on your guard and vigilant in managing your insomnia, and secondly to save yourself from the awful disappointment when the next sleepless night descends.

What do we crave?
Sleep.

What do we want?
A cure. And preferably an instant one. We know it doesn't exist, but that doesn't stop us from seeking one – endlessly.

Dominic's story – the anarchic insomniac
A nice story to finish this chapter on. Dominic, 35, works in PR and is one of life's archetypal owls. So much so he has spent his life hating beds (he refused to have one in his first flat, and bought an eight-foot sofa instead), thinking that beds are a waste of space, and having to go to bed to sleep a total waste of time. His 'cure' is similarly idiosyncratic.

The 'silliness' which is my insomnia happened on Sunday nights. I dreaded going to bed, because I dreaded the fact that I knew I wouldn't be able to go to sleep, and when I did I tossed and turned all night long, chucking the towel in at a disgustingly early 4 a.m. The dread started building as soon as darkness fell, and got progressively worse as the evening wore on. I knew it was my fault, and felt guilty for the fact that I was being silly. Especially when I knew that I was self-perpetuating the misery because at the weekend, to recover from having to get up early during the week to go to work, I'd lay in bed on Saturdays and

Sundays until noon and then feel bad because I'd wasted my precious free time.

On Sunday nights I have a pint of Guinness and a scotch at about 10.30 in the pub over the road, and take a scotch to bed with me to get me off to sleep. I often snack at about 11.30 p.m. – kidneys on toast are my particular tipple, and generally read and scribble myself to sleep – which comes at about 1 or 2 a.m.

Relief came from the most unlikely source: our first baby. Having to get up for her every two hours broke the cycle and meant it wasn't my fault anymore. It also meant I got three shots of unbroken sleep – unheard of! Even better, now the baby sleeps through the night, and so do I. I still read until 1 a.m., but then sleep through until 6 a.m. Nirvana.

Progress: This is probably the first recorded case of babies solving rather than creating sleep problems. Nine months later, Dom is still snoozing well, even on Sunday nights. He gave up drink for a while (which didn't affect his sleep), still suffers resentment about sleep and still sees bed as an inconvenience, but figures this is a personality trait rather than a 'somniacal phenomena'. Anyone else for babies?

z z z z

Our sleeping partners

Insomnia is a single person's disorder. How often we wish we were on our own and could organize our lives as selfishly as we need to give us the space to do all the things to help ourselves get better. Advice about when you eat, what you eat, how you relax, what you do and don't do in the evening – all of it becomes infinitely more complicated when there are two or more to consider. Living with someone adds to the burden, often creating huge strains for both. However supportive your partner may try to be, seeing someone at their worst for much of the time is hardly a recipe for a happy, harmonious domestic life.

Having children to consider as well is an added complication. Family relationships are never easy at the best of times, and adding insomnia into the mix makes normal family life impossible at times. How many insomniac mothers, for example, beat themselves up for being irritable with their children?

Insomniacs can at least confide in each other: your sleeping partner (and children) have to put up with it and, even if they sleep, they suffer the daily side-effects that sleep-deprivation causes. In short, when insomnia hits hard, you get the guilt but they get the misery full on.

It would be wrong to pretend that insomnia causes intolerable burdens in every case. That's not true at all: I know one couple, for example, who are both insomniacs and blissfully happy together. But I absolutely believe that managing your insomnia or sleep-deprivation in the context of the people you love is as important as tackling the demon itself – and deserves its own shout. Sleep books naturally focus on the insomniac, and usually deal with insomnia in isolation. It's as if the people you share your life with either don't exist, or are at best incidental. The reality for many of us is very different. Having insomnia is like having an uninvited, wholly unwelcome and unpleasant guest in your home. I am also reminded of Princess Diana's famous phrase when she said, of her marriage to Prince Charles, that there were three in her marriage, and that made it very crowded. That's certainly what insomnia has felt like for me.

Every relationship is unique, and it is the dynamics of how people who are bound to each other, often in unfathomable ways, which makes it so. It therefore follows that everyone must find their own solution *vis à vis* insomnia as to how to manage the relationships that count most in their life. This isn't a cop-out, just common sense. The purpose of this chapter is to give you a helping hand and some real-life tips for how you might begin.

Partners: how to start

Coping with insomnia tends to creep up on us and our partners; before you know where you are, despite all your good intentions, bad habits and misunderstandings can become the norm. The sooner you can be honest with each other, and the sooner you can adopt an almost workmanlike approach to managing the effects of insomnia – and its potential solutions – the better.

You do need to talk: about how you feel when it's really bad, about whether whatever cure you're trying is working or not, and especially about any changes you want to make to your domestic routine. For example, as an insomniac you may decide arbitrarily that you want to change your diet. You are not going to drink any more wine or eat any more meat; you are going to eat your main meal before 6 p.m. In short, henceforth, all pleasure is to be cancelled, and you will become an oat-loving hermit. Your partner may not like the sound of this at all.

Moving into another bedroom can be dynamite if not handled sensitively. Seemingly trivial things, too, can often cause intense

z z z z

friction, like turning the TV or CD down when you go to bed (because you need quiet), needing the light on (because you need to read) or off (because you need it to be dark), or changing from a duvet to blankets. All these impact just as much on your partner as on you.

Ideally, rather than deciding unilaterally this is what you must do, talk it through first, so both of you feel you're part of the solution.

Is it insomnia or the relationship?

There is no doubt that often insomnia is due, at least in part, to existing strains in a relationship. If so, the sooner you acknowledge these, the better. However hard and however much effort it takes, for both of your sakes you need to be able to separate the insomnia and the difficulties that it causes from the rest of your relationship. In short, don't bring the baggage of what's wrong with your relationship into the insomnia arena, otherwise it'll spell disaster and only make things worse.

To embrace or ignore it?

One of the perennial dilemmas your partner will face is whether to embrace your insomnia – let you talk about it, moan about it, dissect last night's bad sleep at breakfast, etc. – or whether to ignore it as best they can and do their utmost to treat you as 'normal'. My husband and I have tried both. A good rule of thumb is to go by what you (the insomniac) look like in the morning. Most partners will be able to tell at a glance whether it's been a good night or a bad one. When it's bad, someone needs to say something. At such times, hugs are the best and easiest medicine, and will miraculously make things much better.

Richard's Story – Living with an Insomniac

Richard's wife is an insomniac. It rules her life, and hence his. They've done everything but haven't managed to crack it – yet. No prizes for guessing who his wife might be.

z z z z

The worst thing about living with an insomniac for me is the sheer obsessiveness about it which clouds and dominates everything. It seems that insomnia becomes the focus of an insomniac's life to the exclusion of everything else – and it's really difficult to know how to help untie that knot, let alone cope with the fall-out of everyday existence together. Being patient and supportive simply isn't enough, but it's very difficult to know what else to do. Take what to say in the morning, for example. No matter what you say, it never seems to be the right thing.

Having someone else's insomnia disrupt your own sleep is also especially frustrating. If your partner can be calm, that's OK, but the persistent restlessness and tossing and turning through the night can be very wearing.

The thing that would help most is the most obvious: if only your sleepless partner could stop worrying about it so much, it would take a huge amount of pressure off the situation. It's the same with anything in life: if you let it dominate your life, it gets totally out of proportion, which makes it worse for all concerned. Not worrying about it so much, therefore, has to be the first step on the road to recovery.

I understand it better now, and feel immensely sympathetic but also helpless. Over time, I've learned that showing affection is probably the best medicine I can administer. It's certainly what my wife appreciates most.

Owls vs Larks

This is so obvious, but owls and larks do not make the best bed partners, and much avoidable disharmony can be caused by simply not realizing that your partner is an owl while you are a lark, or vice versa. He/she needs to understand that staying up is not your thing; you need to understand that for him/her, going to bed early is like going to bed in the middle of the day. If you both sleep OK, clashing body-clocks are not a major problem. If one of you is an insomniac, it often is. Research in the Netherlands has shown that partners with mismatched sleep patterns have less well-adjusted marriages. Next time, remember to ask first.

ZZ z^Z

Snoring vs Insomnia

One of life's ironies is that, as we get older, women sleep less well and are more prone to insomnia, and men snore more. The two are incompatible. Snorers behave like insomniacs, and believe they don't snore half as much or as loudly as they do, which doesn't help.

It's too much to ask an insomniac to cope with a snoring partner. Persistent loud snoring is a well-known sleep disorder in itself – the snorer needs to seek treatment. If the snoring is not *that* bad, one option is to try products that ease snoring, such as Neversnore™ or Snoreeze (page 257). The insomniac needs to go sleep next door, or to invest in some high-tech earplugs (page 104).

Separate bedrooms

We live in a culture that says being together means sleeping together. As a consequence, sharing the same bed with someone you love is loaded with symbolism both for the sharers and society at large. Irrespective of the reality, it's the most potent, visible sign that you have a happy, harmonious, compatible relationship – and that you have sex. It is also true that a sure sign of an ailing relationship is when you stop sharing the same bed. Speak to marriage guidance councillors or mediators and the statistics overwhelmingly show that when two people stop sleeping together, separation or divorce is on the cards for most couples. Marriages are made in bed, separations are made in the room next door.

Against this background, the very obvious, sensible, grown-up and pragmatic solution to coping with insomnia – which is to start sleeping in your own bedroom, so that you don't disturb your partner, and your partner doesn't disturb you, and all the friction this causes (only saints can be civilized in the middle of the night) – becomes a huge emotional trauma. Your partner feels abandoned, you feel guilty, you both worry whether this is the thin end of the wedge, there is a niggling sense of shame and anxiety about what everyone else will think, and, hell, what about the sex?

The frustrating thing is it doesn't have to be this way. Once the honeymoon is over, fewer people than you think actually make good bedfellows. For example, the recent worldwide sleep survey (see www.neuronic.com) found that a third of the 12,000 people who replied said they were woken up by their partners, 12 per cent by sheet stealing(!) and 15 per cent by snoring and restlessness. One clinical study also showed that sleeping solo is more restful than sleeping *a deux*.

The culture of sleeping together is as much history as emotion – wealthy people have historically had their own separate bedrooms; it's only the rest of us who had to slum it with someone else. The poorer you were, the more people you shared a bed with.

Though it does take adjusting to, in the context of insomnia having separate rooms can help save and nurture a relationship. It is how the two of you *see it* that counts most. I started sleeping in the spare room out of desperation – not a good idea. Much better for *both* of you is to think of it as a safety net, a wonderful bonus and resource which allows you both some respite. A place to go in the middle of the night, if either of you need to, or to begin the night in, or whatever settles as the best pattern for you. Nor do you have to spend all night without each other. A cuddle in the morning works just as well as a cuddle at night.

The only really important thing is that you build in some intimacy. Maintaining physical contact is vital. Putting up with each other's infuriating bedtime habits is not. If in the long term you find you both *prefer* sleeping in separate rooms, so be it. Royals and the rich and privileged have been doing just that for centuries.

Big beds

You can tell how posh and prestigious a hotel is by the size of its beds. But having a big bed is about more than prestige. It makes very good sense. The longer you live with someone, the larger the bed you are likely to need in order for you not to disturb each other's sleep. Going king-size could do wonders for both of you.

zzz z

Sex

By avoiding the subject, or airily saying 'Reserve the bedroom for sleep and sex,' books on insomnia reinforce the myth that your sex life doesn't suffer. It does. There may be a few people in the world this doesn't apply to – teenagers and twenty-somethings or over-sexed males and females come to mind – but for most of us, unless you've just fallen in love, when you can't sleep anyway, your libido takes a nosedive when you have insomnia.

It depends on your personal circumstances and age, but let's be frank, when you're seriously sleep-deprived, 'nosedive' is putting it mildly. Getting it up is not what is in your brain. To quote Paul Martin, in the latest blockbuster on sleep, *Counting Sheep*, 'A tired person can be physically present but psychologically and emotion-ally absent.' You bet.

For normal people, sex before sleep is usually reckoned to be a good sleeping aid. I'm not so sure that's true, let alone for insomni-acs. Arousal is not exactly a passive activity, and sex can wake you up as much as it can relax you. Apparently, this is more so for women. Maybe that's because, as we suspected all along, men are from Mars and women are from Venus. Scientists have also tried testing whether or not orgasms bring on sleep, but without much luck.

There is one truism, however: Use it or lose it. It *is* all too easy when you are knackered not to bother. This doesn't matter for a short time. Nor do you need to make love to someone to have a fulfilling and loving relationship, but generally speaking, for the majority of us, sex is a good idea, at least some of the time. The problem is that the more you *don't* bother, the less you are inclined *to* bother.

The solution is to build your sex life around the times when both of you are awake, not when one of you is desperately seeking sleep. Whatever else you get up to is your business.

Dos and don'ts

If you are an insomniac

- Remember that often your partner needs as much support as you do. Show your appreciation when you can.
- Don't let insomnia rule both of your lives. That's not fair to either of you.
- Try and be less obsessive, and more chilled out. Take a long-term view: it will get better eventually.
- Be nice to yourself. Don't beat yourself up or blame yourself for not sleeping. If you are nice to yourself, you will be much nicer to be around.
- Tossing and turning is usually more disruptive to most partners than reading in bed, or getting out of bed. Train yourself to be poker-still, or go next door.

If your partner is an insomniac

- Don't tell us we had more sleep last night than we say. It doesn't help, especially when it's true. For us, the amount we think we've slept is our reality.
- Don't tell us not to be obsessive. It only aggravates us more.
- Be supportive about lifestyle changes such as diet and exercise. These can really make a difference in many cases, so it's in your interest to give them an opportunity to work. The same goes for relaxation therapies, however bizarre. If your insomniac partner needs to start chanting mantras at odd times of the day or night, or stand motionless outside in the cold for half an hour at midnight practising Chi Kung, so be it. Console yourself that mantras have a calming effect on brain waves, and being still helps you discover yourself. Maybe you should try it, too?
- The nearer you can be a saint, the better. Eventually we'll love you more, promise.
- TLC goes an awful long way. If we need to crawl into bed, or sleep in a different room, tuck us up nicely and whisper sweet nothings in our ear.

z z z z

For both of you

- Physical contact and mutual support are important.
- Hugs work wonders and are the instant, easy way to make things more bearable. Do hugs as often as you can. Remember, there is no such thing as a bad hug – only good ones and great ones.

Jenny's story – on being a saint (for partners only)

Jenny lives with an insomniac – and has wings.

Do take your sleepless partner's condition seriously and appreciate that for them it may be/seem the most important thing in their life and affects everything they do and think.

Do understand that their lack of communication and negativity do not originate with you, nor are they really aimed at you, but sometimes you'll get it in the neck 'cos you're there and your partner can be irritable with you more easily than with friends/colleagues.

Do try and appreciate how desperate, isolated, fragile and vulnerable an insomniac can feel. At the same time, try and help them see things more positively and objectively.

Do understand that insomniacs can become like hermits. Socializing can become a pain rather than a pleasure. You may find you have to undertake more social outings or other activities on your own, but always talk about it rather than letting a gulf open up.

Do encourage – without badgering – your partner to work at handling the effects of insomnia and working at improving the amount of sleep they get. If you have an interest, help them look for potential remedies: books, counsellors, sleep clinics, etc.

Do try and be accommodating if your partner feels it necessary to develop a bedtime ritual, such as going to bed early/late, doing meditation, primal screaming, reading in bed or going off to try and sleep in the spare room.

Don't encourage them to obsess about their condition. Help nurture peace and tranquillity rather than anxiety and brooding.

Don't debate anything controversial with your partner late at night. Agree to discuss it earlier in the day, or wait until the next day.

Don't put your own sleep at risk by adopting or allowing yourself to be overly disrupted by your partner's routine. It will make you irritable and them guilty. And two insomniacs are definitely not better than one.

Don't say 'You're ruining my life/your life/our lives/our holiday.' They will already be aware of this if this is the case, and often feel all the more angry and frustrated with themselves because of it.

Don't say 'You got more sleep than you think.' Even if this were true, which usually it is not, remember that it is the subjective experience of the insomniac that matters.

Don't say you had a bad night too, just because you only got seven hours instead of your usual eight. Missing the odd hour or two occasionally is not the same as only getting two or three hours for nights on end.

Don't accuse them of not being romantic, affectionate or positive. It's hard to be anything other than a shadow if you haven't slept for weeks.

z z z z

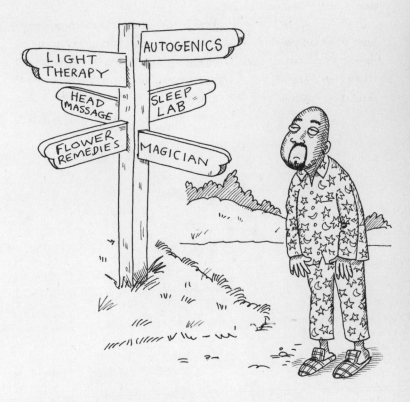

PART 3

Getting it sorted

Before we begin ...

Understanding insomnia or not being able to sleep well, and the way it impinges on you, your life and the life of your loved ones, is one thing; doing something about it is quite another. I am always surprised, for example, at the number of insomniacs I talk to who basically have never really bothered to do anything about their lack of sleep. I cannot say why (it's different for everyone), but I think inertia plays a big part – or rather that the effort involved seems insurmountable. Sleep specialists find the same.

For it is EFFORT that is the key. I learned the hard way that managing insomnia requires personal effort and discipline. You have to own and take responsibility for your insomnia, and have the will to change your habits and, sometimes, your life. Sounds crazy maybe, but just think of how much effort it takes to relax, let alone find a method of relaxation that works for you and that you can stick at. What we need is a Weight Watchers or Alcoholics Anonymous equivalent for insomnia – local clubs where we can share our despair and follow a pre-determined path to recovery. What we get is 'absent healing' in the form of books. I have quite a collection myself. They all make good sense, they all give excellent advice, many promise a cure, sometimes in days – and I haven't yet stuck at any of them. Why? Because you have to do it all by yourself. And that's the hardest thing of all. Sleep-disorder centres and clinics provide an infrastructure of support, but the rest of us muddle on in isolation.

This is not to say you don't need props, medical help or some magic from your favourite healer. You need these as well. But unless you're very lucky, or your insomnia or poor sleep is due to a simple external cause, moving forward means management. For me, it's one of the biggest lessons I've learned. I can't pretend that digging deep and finding the quiet determination to change your attitude comes easy, but you can at least take it at your own pace. I'm also absolutely convinced it's the first step on the road to recovery. The reward? The promise of better sleep and a better you.

Insomnia in a nutshell

The *Sivananda Book of Meditation* makes the point that meditation, like sleep, cannot be taught: It's something you just fall into. Which is what sleep scientists such as Dr Adrian Williams, Consultant Physician at St Thomas' Hospital, confirms:

The harder we try to sleep, the less we are able to sleep. Sleep only comes when we don't really care. Arousal takes precedence over sleep. In a conflict between the need to sleep and the need to stay aroused, arousal usually wins. To be able to sleep, we need to feel safe and slightly bored. The time course for arousal is rapid, of relaxation slow. Once we are aroused, it may take many minutes to slowly calm down again. Insomniacs are adept at creating and internalizing threats. Things that others can set aside and worry about tomorrow, the insomniac has to take care of before sleeping. The longer insomnia lasts, the worse it gets because perpetuating factors come into play and the initial factors may no longer be important.

Although a principal cause of insomnia can be found [in one of] five categories -- medical, psychiatric, drug, behavioural, and circadian rhythm disorders -- more often than not more than one cause is operative in maintaining the inability to get to sleep or to stay asleep.

z z z z

The Master Plan: Essentials

There are lots of things you can do to encourage, improve and nurture good sleep. If your sleeping problems are recent, something simple like a few judicious lifestyle changes may be all you need – or at least make the difference that counts to enable improvement. Long-term insomniacs are different. We are tough nuts to crack, and there is no point pretending otherwise. I have had (and still have) too many false sleepless dawns to believe anyone who tells me otherwise. This does not mean there is no hope. Quite the reverse. But it does mean you need to trawl the various 'remedies' and sleep strategies until you find the individual combination that works for you, and to be rigorous about employing them until that wonderful day arrives when thinking about sleep is yesterday's story.

I have also resisted the '10-day cure approach' – which isn't to say they don't work for some people (and may work for you) – just that they haven't worked for me. Three years into this game I understand that the path to resolving chronic or persistent insomnia is neither straight nor easy, and takes time and dedication to follow. Miracles apart, it is not something you cure overnight.

Looking back on my own history of trying (and often failing) to cope with insomnia, I understand much better the mistakes I have made. The big one, of course, is thrashing around trying this and that and anything out of desperation, starting with a mixture of supplements and ricocheting from one therapist to the next, everyone from sleep specialists to spiritual healers. The battle has at least given me more insight into what needs to be done, and how the steps are interlinked.

The Master Plan offers an integrated approach which I fervently believe is the best way to tackle insomnia or serious sleep problems. It's a prescription for good sleep. If I had followed it a year or so ago, I know I would have saved myself a lot of grief; my aim is to save you from some of yours.

This is how one insomniac sees it:

To me there are causes of insomnia and excuses for it – I tend to focus on the latter. If there are a number of causes and some are removed, then I think that those that remain may even be amplified – to make things worse. I'm also sure that the more I think about not sleeping, the less that I do. I believe there are initial trigger points of insomnia which are latent in all of us and then triggered. Recognition of the initial trigger must therefore be key to its cure. It then becomes a learned behaviour and then much more difficult to cure.

I think that personal ownership and intuition are keys to which path a person should take. I have a clear metaphorical image in my head of water following a journey down a mountainside. It meets many block-ages and diversions and becomes quite muddy. The dirty reduced flow reduces my ability to sleep. It is my challenge to remove the blockages and the 'dirt' so there is a clear path through. I can get sufficient sleep from the current flow, but will only achieve the seven hours by putting in more work.

– Barry

The heart of the matter

Having lived, breathed and thought of insomnia and little else for some time now, I have come to the conclusion that sleeping pill dependency apart (see page 205), ordinary insomnia and not being able to sleep generally break down into three core conditions, and consequently you need a three-pronged attack:

1. *Stress:* You need to get your cortisol levels down and serotonin levels up.
2. *Dysfunctional sleep pattern/body-clock:* You need to re-programme your sleep patterns, get your body-clock back on course, coax your body/mind into better sleep and re-learn normal sleeping patterns.
3. *Fixing the software:* You need to unlearn all those negative thoughts and behaviours about not being able to sleep.

The Master Plan

Preliminaries

Phase 1: The easy stuff

Phase 2: Tackling stress

Phase 3: Getting further help

The Master Plan is designed to give you the big picture. It gives you structure and focus so you can identify which steps you need most to tackle and, equally important, to be honest with yourself about it.

z z z z

All of the steps outlined above are linked. You are going to have to address all of them to a certain degree, but some will be more important for your insomnia than others.

You need certain basics in place before you can move on to the next step. For example, sorting your sleep hygiene and diet are fundamental prerequisites to improving sleep. So make sure this is in place first.

Some of the steps inevitably work in tandem – as everyone is different, you will have to decide which order is likely to be best for you. If your mind doesn't work like this (my mind is irrevocably anarchic and can never follow someone else's set pattern for more than five minutes), then just start at the top and work your way down. If it's worked for me, it should work for you.

You're aiming to equip yourself with your own personal tool-kit for managing and promoting better sleep. (Actually, you're secretly aiming for a cure, but no point raising expectations yet.) Like any tool-kit, expect to add new items as you find them, and chuck out old redundant ones when they no longer do the job as effectively. Variety is the key.

Do whatever feels right, but do it. And make sure you triumphantly tick the steps off as you do.

Questions to ask yourself

- Is your insomnia or poor sleep something that is primarily to do with a bad bedroom, and/or diet and lifestyle habits?
- Is it primarily a physiological, medical, emotional or psychological problem?
- Is it primarily causing you stress, or is stress causing your insomnia?

Cardinal sins

- Never go to bed angry and don't get involved in arguments before you go to bed. Anger is a destructive

z z z z

emotion, and causes cortisol hormones to be released which will prevent you from getting to sleep. Don't get angry with yourself or your insomnia during the night either. If you do nothing else, learn to be at peace with your insomnia during the night.

- Don't drink yourself to sleep. It doesn't work. You may crash out initially, but alcohol will exacerbate your insomnia and you will pay for it in the middle of the night.
- Don't drink caffeine before you go to bed, or after 2 p.m. at the latest. It makes your brain buzz, raises your heart rate and puts your system on red alert.
- Don't smoke. If you can't kick the habit, cut down as much as you can and give up smoking in the evening.

Dos and Don'ts

- Give yourself a break, and stop dreaming about 8 hours' perfect sleep. Not that many people achieve this. Reduce your expectations about how much sleep you ideally want and you will begin to feel much better.
- Be honest and work out how much sleep you need to be able to function. You may find it's less than you want or hope for. Anything else then becomes a bonus rather than an unfulfilled right.
- Unless you are a masochist, do skip chapters in books on insomnia and sleep on the horrors that sleep-deprivation causes. It only adds to your overall anxiety levels – and it is anxiety, rather than lack of sleep, that you should be worried about.

Preliminaries

What kind of sleeper are you?

All other things being equal, your basic natural sleeping pattern is conditioned by whether you are an owl or lark and a naturally

z z z z

short- or long-sleeper. Use the information on pages 16 and 9 to work this out first, before you begin to do anything else, as it provides you with the basic framework within which your insomnia or poor sleeping habits have to be tackled. For example, if you are naturally a short-sleeper, you don't need eight hours' sleep so there's no point hoping or aiming for it. Remember when trying to assess whether you are a short or long sleeper that most of us tend to gravitate to shorter sleeping as we get older, so what might have been true 20 years ago is not necessarily true now. Similarly, if you are an owl, adopting sleep-restriction practices or behavioural modifications that suit larks will be a struggle at best, and a waste of time at worst.

What kind of insomnia do you have, and what kind of insomniac are you?

The kind of insomnia you have, and the kind of insomniac you are, are also starting points and hold valuable clues as to how to approach taming it. Use the information on page 56 to help you work this out. You will also need to fill in a sleep diary for one week (or two).

Also, your view of what kind of insomniac you are *should* be personal. This is not an exercise to label you, but an exercise in being honest with yourself and the probable causes of your insomnia. It's only by rigorously examining these, as well as yourself, that you can begin to home in on the real problems, and therefore begin to prioritize them. It also means you don't have to worry about aspects that don't relate to you.

Once you have accomplished this, you can take a look at the other elements in the Master Plan, step by step and chapter by chapter, beginning with 'The Easy Stuff', next.

z z z z

Phase One:
The easy stuff

This is the really basic, easy bit everyone can do to help themselves get a better night's sleep, and there's no excuse not to address these.

Sleep hygiene

This rather bizarre sleep term means making sure that your sleep environment is conducive to sleep rather than hindering or preventing it.

Beds and pillows

Your bed is the most important sleep tool you have, and too many of us do not pay enough attention to it, or spend enough money on it or on the pillows we rest our heads on for a third of our lives. Investing in a first-class bed is a life-enhancing investment. For the sleep-deprived, it is a must. Research has shown that simply by changing from an uncomfortable bed to a comfortable one, people sleep longer and toss and turn less: in a comfortable bed you may move around 20–30 times a night in your sleep; in an uncomfortable bed this can shoot up to 100 times a night. As a rough rule of thumb, the firmer the bed (which does *not* mean the harder), the better. Native Americans used to sleep with their backs against trees. Think about it – just try lying on your back on the floor, and see how amazingly restful and calming it is. Not that many of us ever stay still in one position long enough, but orthopaedically the best position to sleep in is either on your back or side; for calmer sleep, the right side is believed to be best.

For where to start on buying beds, the industry-funded Sleep Council *Bed-Buyers Guide* spells out the basics (available on-line at: www.sleepcouncil.com or tel. 01756 792 327).

A pillow is just as important (did you know that your head accounts for 20 per cent of your body weight?) Forget advice on what pillow or how many you should have; it's what suits you that counts. I know, I've tried them all from the softest to the most orthopaedically challenging. And remember that the average life of a mattress is 10 years, a pillow 2 years.

The quality of your bed linen also counts, especially if you get sweaty. Natural fabrics are best. These days there's a good choice of organic bed linen, too. Avoiding allergens (especially house mites), which hinder breathing, is important for some people: Yorkwellbeing (www.homeinonhealth.com) supply home kits and house dust mite home check kits and anti-allergy bedding. Don't forget that some people find tucking a pillow under or between their legs a sleep-inducing comforter.

In the West we sleep on mattresses. Some people swear by futons or hammocks, others by water beds, which have grown up and become respectable – they can feel strange at first to those of us used to something more inflexible, but there is no denying their calming effect. The British Waterbed Company (www.waterbed.co.uk) is the place to start. In America, water pillows are promoted to relieve neck and head pain and to promote more restful sleep. See, for example, www.pillowrx.com.

Bed position

Which way your bed (and therefore your head) faces, and where it is in the bedroom, may matter more than you think. This is because the earth's electromagnetic fields, and which way they run in your bedroom, have subtle effects which may affect your sleep. Geopathic stress – the natural and artificial electromagnetic forces that surround us – is real enough, and if you are sleeping over a

z z z z

geo-pathic zone it can disturb your sleep (and your health). Charles Dickens worked this out and always slept with his head facing north, so that the currents would flow through his body and enhance his sleep. You can ask a professional dowser or kinesiologist to find the best position for you, or work it out using Feng Shui principles. As for the rest of your bedroom, it goes without saying that to promote restful sleep, your bedroom should be simple, decorated in soothing pastel colours, and be *uncluttered.*

For magnetic therapy, magnet pillows and mattresses, see page 171. For the Ayurvedic way, see page 217.

Feng Shui bedroom savvy

Feng Shui harmonizes *chi* (energy) in your environment to your best advantage. This means it's not just which way you face that matters (determined according to the Pa Kua chart, which sets out the most propitious way you should face, according to your birthdate – and can make a real difference sleepwise for some people), but the shape of the room, how the furniture is arranged, what kind of furniture it contains (mirrors are taboo), where it is in relation to the stairs and bathroom, and so on. Not only that, you have to clap out any trapped, stagnant *chi.* It all makes very good sense but would take many pages to explain it all, so for once I am going to suggest you do the research for yourself. *Learn to Sleep Well* gives you the bones (and a Pa Kua chart). The *Illustrated Encyclopedia of Feng Shui* does bedrooms comprehensively. Or call in a Feng Shui expert who will do the job for you.

Peace and quiet

Noise definitely disturbs sleep, particularly REM sleep. It is fact, not fiction, that people sleep better in a quiet location. This means your bedroom should be peaceful and quiet. No TV, phone or computer, ticking clock or the faint noise of a dripping gutter that you've been meaning to do something about. If you live on a main road, move into the back bedroom if you can. Do not work in bed; the most you are allowed is a little light and pleasant reading matter – or, if you feel up to it, sex. Snoring partners are a no-no. You need to set up your own little sleep nest in a different room – or do earplugs big time.

Sounds you like (see page 170) that make you feel safe, secure and snug, such as soothing music, the sounds of the ocean, etc., are different. They can be used to mask unwelcome sounds or just lull you to sleep.

Earplugs

If you can't do anything about noise, try earplugs. I find cheap ones immensely uncomfortable, but they do reduce noise levels by up to 50 per cent. You have a choice of foam that you squeeze first and put in your ears, which then expands to fill your ear cavity, or wax, both available from chemists (and free on many long-haul flights). They feel peculiar, but are cheap.

Elacin sleepfits

This is the other alternative. A small specialist hearing-protection company (Advanced Communication Solutions Ltd) produce sophisticated custom-made earmoulds for musicians, motorcyclists, shift workers, etc., not to mention Formula One racing drivers. For sleep they use the strongest filter and softest silicon material. The Sleepfits are dinky and work very well at reducing noise levels, including that from snoring partners. I found them fiddly to put in at first, but am very pleased with mine. They last at least five years, and are worth the investment if noise is an issue in your life. No guarantees (or money back, obviously, though they will refund the cost of the filter, which is almost half), but if noise is the cause of your insomnia it may crack the problem. They come in very useful for long plane flights, noisy mowers and strimmers, also. To obtain them you first need to see one of their accredited audiologists (located in the UK and worldwide) who will take an impression of both ears, which is then used to make your personal set of Sleepfits. Get the audiologist to show you how to put them in properly (easy once you've been shown how). At the time of writing they cost around £90. For details see page 252 or visit www.hearingprotection.co.uk.

z z z z

Light and temperature

Your bedroom should be dark – invest in heavy curtains that exclude light or that have blackout linings, or buy some blackout blinds (see www.blinds.co.uk). If you can't do this, sleep with an eye mask. Sadly there are precious few really user-friendly ones out there; it's the thin pieces of elastic that are the really annoying and uncomfortable bit. Make sure the mask is thick enough and frames enough of your face to exclude the light. Those offered on long-haul flights are not bad.

For the lovely lavender eye-pillow, see page 165.

For tips on bright light therapy, see page 194.

Temperature has a huge effect on how well you are likely to sleep. Not too hot and not too cold is the maxim, or around 62°F (16°C) or a little warmer for the bedroom. A baby's room should be kept at around 65°F (18°C). And you may find it a pain and a shame, but you should switch to blankets which you can put on or take off rather than a duvet. This also allows you to cope better with your own body temperature, which changes according to your biological body-clock, irrespective of how hot or cold your bedroom is.

Though it doesn't feel like it for those of us who wake up boiling hot in the middle of the night, we are designed to be warmest early evening, then gradually cool off as the evening advances, becoming coldest at about 3.30–4 a.m. In other words, keep your bedroom cool when you go to bed and during the night, and time the central heating to come on after dawn. As for your duvet, one sleep-deprived friend passed me on this tip which her chiropracter advised: put your duvet under the sheet and sleep *on* it, not under it. It worked for her.

Clocks

A digital clock that makes no noise, has BIG numbers that you can see easily and which has an illuminator at the touch of a finger is what you need. Most sleep experts advise against clock-watching; this makes very good sense. As a general rule, *don't* look at the clock. Keep it turned away from you so you can't see what time it is unless you make a positive attempt to do so. Occasionally it can help – especially when it gives you a nice surprise and it's nearer morning than you thought. Just be aware that it is just as likely to be earlier than you hoped for, so *only* look if you are prepared for this and can promise yourself you won't get into a tizz. If this happens, do an instant double-take and console yourself that the night is young and you still have ample opportunity to sleep.

Routine

Very boring, but developing a routine is sacrosanct. All sleep scientists are adamant about this: wherever possible, go to bed at the same time, and always get up at the same time. It's called re-training your brain. You won't succeed 100 per cent, but the closer you can get to this, the better it bodes for your sleep. For more on this, see page 198.

Being secure

Feeling safe and secure in bed is important. Our ancestors were primed to be on the look-out, so feeling vulnerable when we sleep is inbuilt. Modern life brings its fair share of threats in the night – being burgled, for instance, as happened to Will (page 65), which threw his insomnia into overdrive, being an obvious one. Sleeping in a house on your own, especially if you are a woman, can be disconcerting, as I know well. This isn't an issue for everyone, but if it is for you, making sure your environment is physically safe is important.

z z z z

Wind-down time

Winding down before you go to bed is like foreplay: we don't always bother but it makes an awful lot of difference. Every insomniac I've spoken to confirms this. Our sleep needs to be treated with kid gloves, especially around bedtime. The golden rules are:

- Take time to go to bed, and try and go to bed at the same time every night.
- Get today out of your head: write out the day's events, or what you have to do tomorrow, in a worry book if you need to.
- Don't argue, watch violent TV, listen to Beethoven's 7th, play games, get on the computer, pay bills or watch movies just before you go to bed.
- Choose a cuddle over a stimulating bed-time chat every time.
- A hot bath is the easy and pleasurable way to relax. Add whatever relaxing potions you like. Just remember to take it an hour or more before you go to bed. Or try my version (page 147).

Eating to sleep

I have spent my life believing absolutely that you are what you eat. Nutrition for life – and now, sleep – remains one of my consuming passions. How much changing your diet can improve your sleep, however, depends on what your diet was like in the first place, your particular bio-foibles (are you the one-in-a-million who can consume a large tub of ice-cream at 1 a.m. and still drop right off?) and the underlying cause of your sleeplessness. As an insomniac, I also find advice such as eating an open turkey and cottage cheese sandwich or a banana (or both) just before you go to bed a bit divorced from real life. Does anyone actually want to do this? But I do believe

– and there is certainly more than enough evidence around – that making changes to your diet can help foster good sleep.

You need to tackle this in two ways: getting rid of the eating habits that prevent good sleep, and substituting habits and foods that will help promote it.

Before you begin, a piece of advice picked up in *Seven Days to a Perfect Night's Sleep*: write down what and when you eat and drink in your sleep diary for a week, and see if there are any correlations between your diet and sleep patterns. You can then start by eliminating potential trouble-makers. You'll probably find, like one sleepless friend, that however much you like them, late-night pizzas will just have to go.

Bad sleep diets

As we all know, Friday night vindaloos washed down with several lagers are not the recipe for sleep; nor is tucking into your favourite cheese at midnight (cheese contains a substance called tyramine, which indirectly leads to an increase in blood pressure, a symptom associated with nightmares). Foods which are difficult or take a long time to digest, high-sugar foods which take no time to digest but which give the body and brain a rush of fuel, too much alcohol and caffeine, foods containing the additive MSG (monosodium glutamate, found in many processed foods and take-aways) which causes, among other things, digestive problems, headaches and heartburn, foods and drinks containing the yellow peril, tartrazene (E-102), notorious for its link with hyperactivity in children – all of these can negatively affect your sleep. Life as an insomniac is already miserable enough. Cut them out or reduce them as much as you can from your diet.

The other substance nutritionists advise to avoid is aspartame (Nutrasweet). Apart from being a stimulant, it depletes tryptophan and serotonin levels.

As we all know, too, large quantities of fat and protein hang around in the system and are difficult to digest. Both take twice as long (about 4 hours) as carbohydrate to metabolize – another reason to go easy on the butter and cream (or olive oil) in the evening. Furthermore, despite what Mediterraneans do, the digestive system does not work half as well in the evening as during the day.

Other foods to avoid are: processed foods, which are poor-value nutrition and, biologically speaking, just a waste of space; spicy foods – hot spices such as chilli and mustard, which act as stimulants; foods high in tyrosine, especially before bedtime. Tyrosine is an amino acid that increases the release of norepinephrine – the neurotransmitter that does for the brain what adrenaline does for the body. Examples are bacon and other cured meats, aged cheeses such as parmesan, blue cheeses such as Stilton, soft cheeses such as mozzarella, potatoes, tomatoes, chocolate and also wine. Now we know why pizzas and chianti give us a buzz.

Junk food diets are a no-no. So is *not* eating – I've been there myself, when you are literally too tired to eat, and know of other insomniacs who, through stress and anxiety, end up not eating. As far as your body is concerned, both are extremely stressful. If you don't believe me, read *The Mood Cure* by Dr Julia Ross.

The final aspect of your diet worth checking are food allergens: wheat (gluten), dairy, nuts and oranges are among the most common culprits. For help, see Allergy UK, page 265.

All this makes very good sense, but don't go into a panic. It doesn't mean these are banned foods, or that your insomnia will spiral out of control if you have a bacon butty at 9 p.m. You know what you can eat and what you can't. If you don't, this is a very good time to find out. Even if you do nothing else, you can at least become more strategic about when you eat what. Your sleep will thank you for it.

Don't eat large meals close to bedtime; in fact, if you can, ideally aim to eat lightly in the evening, and save binges for lunchtime. At the very least, avoid foods which give your liver a hard time and are difficult to digest. Absolutely avoid any kind of sugar at bedtime in the form of food or drink. It's an instant source of energy for the brain at exactly at the wrong time. Incorporate sleep-friendly foods into your diet. For these see page 110.

Drinking

Don't drink fluids before you go to bed: otherwise you'll have to pee in the middle of the night.

Caffeine, alcohol and nicotine

If you are serious about doing something about your insomnia then you are going to have to significantly – that is, drastically – reduce your intake of these three substances.

- Ideally, cut all three out of your life. If that's not possible, then use them strategically. Be strict with yourself and severely limit your intake – at least most of the time (we make allowances for the fact that we are mortals, not angels).
- Limit alcohol consumption to 1–2 units, and make sure you drink your alcohol well before bedtime. For choice, stay with decent wine rather than beer or spirits. Switch to a glass of hot milk before bedtime: it's just as comforting as a nip of brandy. And try not to drink every night.
- Limit caffeine to 1–2 cups of coffee per day, and always in the morning. Don't drink coffee or strong tea after lunchtime – ideally, you need to allow 10 hours before bedtime to be caffeine-free.
- If you can't give up smoking, reduce it as much as you can, and try not to smoke in the evening (you need at least four hours for the disruptive effects of nicotine to work through your system), and definitely not before you go to bed, or in bed.

Good sleep diets

Good sleep diets are those which avoid overloading the digestion, go easy on the liver, do not cause your blood-sugar levels to yo yo, contain copious quantities of water and maximize key nutrients for sleep – namely B vitamins, calcium and magnesium, zinc and

z z z z

tryptophan. You *don't* need to go mad, but you *do* need regular protein, and regular fat. Junk foods and empty-calorie foods are not on the menu. And I would say this, wouldn't I?, but eat organic when you can. It's the best way to minimize the potential toxic overload from your diet.

Diet is also a factor in stress. Bad diets are themselves very stressful. Good diets, with lots of the good-mood foods discussed here will help to combat the biochemical effects of stress. And good-mood foods are exactly the same as good-sleep foods – another bonus.

What the experts say: food and sleep

There are three main areas where food can have a specific effect on sleep: the use of stimulants, especially caffeine; eating the wrong kind of carbohydrates, namely refined white sugar and starches, which upset blood sugar levels by causing blood sugar levels to rise dramatically and then dip too low; and food intolerances, which, in my experience are more prevalent than the general public or GPs realize. All affect sleep adversely, and can be a cause of insomnia. The other area to consider is multiple-chemical sensitivity. This is more challenging, as it can require major changes to diet, including switching to organic foods, and means that you have to really clean up your act and your environment.

To say this or that in the diet can cure most types of insomnia, however, is too simplistic. It's creating that balance between getting rid of the 'stressors' and increasing the 'supporters', which is why it is important to eat foods with the right sleep-inducing vitamins and minerals, and reinforce this perhaps with a multivitamin and -mineral supplement. Increasing protein can help, as it gets more tryptophan into the system and, importantly, helps to stabilize blood sugar levels – dips during the night are a common cause of waking. The psychological effect of taking control of your diet shouldn't be underestimated, either. It gives people confidence and a boost to their self-worth, and I find with many project participants that this alone is a huge help.

Amanda Geary, Founder of the Food and Mood Project (www.foodandmood.org)

Water

Water is any health spa's favourite cure and detox weapon. The body loses about 1.7–2.3 litres (3–4 pints) of fluid a day, which it needs to make up. A bore, I know, but drinking tea and coffee doesn't count. What you need is water. It stops you from being dehydrated, flushes out the toxins and helps ensure your kidneys and liver are happy, which is what you need if you want to sleep well. Pilots, for example, are advised to drink plenty of water to help with their sleep and jet-lag.

The normal prescription is a large glass of water every hour during the day; given that life isn't perfect, just get as near to this as you can manage. If drinking water is not part of your current lifestyle, give it a try for a week or two (your bladder soon settles down) and see the difference it makes to your well-being – and hopefully your sleep.

Top Tips

Drink still water. It's easier, and carbonated water aggravates the digestive system. Naturally carbonated water is different. Its bubbles come from the fact they are highly mineralized and therefore naturally fizzy. These aid digestion; added carbon dioxide doesn't.

- Always drink from a large glass, at least a half-pint one.
- Buy yourself two 1-litre bottles of still mineral water. Keep them on your work desk, in the kitchen, lounge and bedroom. Make sure you empty one a day.
- Don't drink chilled or iced water. It's more difficult to drink in quantity. Warm it up with a splash of boiling water first, as By contrast, warm water is soothing and easy to drink.
- To vary, add a slice organic lemon or peeled and chopped fresh ginger. It tastes nice, and both are fearsomely good for you.
- Don't forget, start the day with a glass of hot water and slice of lemon. It'll make you feel much better about that lovely cup of coffee you're just about to make.

z z z z

Key nutrients for sleep

The list below shows how easy it is to get these nutrients in your diet, and why you should have them.

B-vitamins

B-vitamins generally are essential for the proper functioning of your nervous and endrocrine systems (the glands that produce hormones), and vital for mental health and memory. They are water soluble, so you need to replenish supplies constantly. Several play an important role in sleep. A lack of them can affect sleep. B-vitamins need other B-vitamins do their job properly, so you need to eat a range of foods to ensure you get a variety, not just the one that's best for sleep, or that you think you may be deficient in. Or opt for a B-complex supplement (taken early in the day, not at night). Alcohol, tea, coffee, smoking, and stress rob you of them.

B6 – Pyridoxine

A vital sleep vitamin. It stimulates the pineal gland to secrete more melatonin, and is required to convert tryptophan into serotonin. A lack of B_6 can also affect your ability to dream and recall dreams.

Good sources

Turbot, wholegrains, wheatgerm, red kidney beans, potatoes, watercress, bananas, dried apricots, walnuts.

B12 – Cobalamin

Thought to be instrumental in the production of melatonin, and helps normalize circadian rhythms. Older people find it more difficult to absorb vitamin B_{12} from food, making them a special case where sleep is concerned; vegans have to work hard to get adequate amounts from their diet.

Good sources

Dairy products, seafood, oysters, eggs, miso, sea vegetables, fortified breakfast cereals.

B₃ – Niacin

Aids transformation of tryptophan into serotonin and has been found to improve REM sleep and decrease waking time during the night. It is also important for mental health.

Good sources

Red meat, chicken and turkey, tuna, salmon, mackerel, fortified breakfast cereals, wholewheat, wheatgerm, mushrooms, dried apricots.

B₅ – Pantothenic acid

Involved in energy-production and helps make anti-stress hormones and the memory-boosting neurotransmitter acetylcholine. Lack of it increases anxiety, is not good for stress – and hence sleep – and reduces dreaming.

Good sources

Meat, brewer's yeast, liver, eggs, wheatgerm, mushrooms, avocados, tomatoes, broad beans, peanuts.

B₁ – Thiamine

Promotes healthy nerves, is a mood-enhancer and also helps metabolize carbohydrates and turn glucose (the brain's fuel) into energy – a deficiency results in mental and physical tiredness. People with insomnia often have low levels of vitamin B_1. Older people are more prone to deficiencies, and it has been shown that extra thiamine can be beneficial for their sleep.

Good sources

Avocados, grains, sunflower seeds, Brazil nuts, pork, salmon, mussels, soy milk.

Calcium and magnesium

Magnesium is known as Nature's calmer. It's a nerve mineral, soothing neuron excitability, and is found in abundant quantities in the brain. Lack of this vital mineral can be a contributory cause of insomnia, while adding therapeutic doses to the diet has been found to reduce the time it takes to get to sleep and the frequency of waking in the night, and relieves daytime anxiety.

Calcium has a similar effect, and has recently been billed by American health expert Robert R Barefoot as the most important mineral for your health, longevity and disease-prevention. It maintains the acid-alkali balance in the body.

Calcium and magnesium work in tandem – both are essential for most physiological processes in the body. There must be sufficient of both available, which is why supplements often combine the two.

Good sources

Magnesium: Avocados, wheatgerm, buckwheat flour, bananas, green leafy vegetables, wholegrains, nuts and seeds, soya, peanut butter.
Calcium: Dairy products, brewer's yeast, corn tortillas, green beans, broccoli, parsley, pumpkin seeds, cooked dried beans, whole sardines, almonds, calcium-enriched soy milk, molasses.

Tryptophan

Tryptophan is an essential amino acid, and the reason insomniacs are told to have a love-in with turkey. Your body converts tryptophan into mood-enhancing serotonin, from which the sleep hormone melatonin is made, and turkey (and chicken) are stuffed full of it. Indeed, tryptophan is found in a wide range of foods – all animal proteins contain it, including that glass of hot milk at bedtime and that magic banana or bowl of porridge – so getting extra is a really easy way to nurture yourself and your sleep.

However, tryptophan only works effectively if there is sufficient carbohydrate in the bloodstream, otherwise other amino acids, which are usually in greater supply, compete with it at the blood/brain barrier, blocking its entry into the brain, which is where serotonin is manufactured. Carbohydrates increase the release of insulin, which binds with other amino acids present, leaving tryptophan a clear run.

Hence the turkey sandwich bit. Though if you do start munching these at bedtime, be sure to use wholewheat bread or crackers, otherwise you'll be in for instant carbo release and the roller-coaster sugar effect that comes from refined carbohydrates, which will wake you up again.

Confusingly, the jury is out on whether you actually need to eat protein and carbohydrate together, or eat them separately. One study in America also found that high carbohydrate caused an increase of brain serotonin on its own; health writer Susan Clark points out, too, that people who eat a wholefood carbohydrate-based diet are found to be calmer, rarely depressed and sleep more soundly. Nutritionists like Dr Julia Ross think carbo cravings in the afternoon and evening or during the night can be the body's way of signalling that it needs more serotonin – and can often be fixed by taking serotonin supplements (see page 125). She also points out that skipping meals or eating meals without protein is almost guaranteed to reduce serotonin, and that people who do not get enough fat in their diet are often moody. Which, I guess, is why gourmets are also often contented and sleep like babies.

Good sources

Meat – especially turkey and chicken, fish – especially tuna and salmon, dairy products – especially cottage cheese and milk, rolled oats, eggs, tofu, wholewheat bread, kidney beans, lentils and chick-peas, pumpkin and sunflower seeds, avocados, figs and dates, bananas, pineapples, spinach, walnuts, peanuts.

Note that alcohol blocks tryptophan.

Babies and tryptophan: Breast milk has a high ratio of tryptophan (around 17 per cent of total protein, or 1.7 g/per 100 g), higher than cow's or soya milk. If your baby is being fed infant formula, double-check its tryptophan content.

z z z z

Sprouts for sleep

Sprouted seeds are a storehouse of vitamins and minerals, and hence one of the easiest ways to cram these into your diet. Bioforce produce the niftiest and best free booklet I have found on how to sprout seeds for yourself. One is *Healthy Sprouts* by Gillian Miller, available from healthfood shops. For aiding sleep, try the following sprouted seeds:

- quinoa (all B vitamins, calcium, all essential amino acids)
- lentils (B_1, B_2, B_3, B_6, B_{12}, vitamin C, zinc)
- alfalfa (magnesium, all essential amino acids)

Tryptophan meals

Each of the following gives you 500 mg tryptophan, and illustrates that good-for-sleep meals are perfectly normal, and simple to make.

- Oat porridge, soya milk and two scrambled eggs
- Baked potato with cottage cheese and tuna salad
- Chicken breast, potatoes au gratin and green beans
- Wholewheat spaghetti with bean, tofu or meat sauce
- Salmon fillet, quinoa and lentil pilaf and green salad with yoghurt dressing

Source: *Optimum Nutrition for the Mind*, by Patrick Holford

Vitamin C

Vital anti-oxidant, strengthens the immune system, helps make anti-stress hormones (the adrenals are gross feeders – see page 121), and used up rapidly if stress is high and sleep is poor.

Good sources

Ripe fruits – especially kiwi, orange, mango, blackcurrants – red peppers, ripe tomatoes.

Zinc

Needed for vitamin B absorption, especially B_6, and a critical element for mental health, yet also the most commonly deficient mineral. Zinc levels fall if stress is high and sleep is poor; a lack of zinc also reduces dream recall.

Good sources

Oysters (the richest source of all), grains, nuts and seeds, meat and fish, egg yolk, ginger.

Silicon

Improves calcium metabolism and strengthens nerve tissue.

Good sources

Cucumber, celery, lettuce, barley.

Inositol

Necessary for cell and nerve growth and regeneration, involved in neurotransmitter function, and reduces blood cholesterol. Insomnia is often a symptom of deficiency.

Good sources

Eggs, fish, liver, wheatgrain, soya, nuts, pulses, lecithin granules, citrus fruits, especially grapefruit.

The best time to eat

Eating provides the body with fuel, raises your metabolic rate and causes your body temperature to rise. This is why you should avoid late-night meals or heavy meals in the evening – you are reversing nature's natural trigger for sleep, which is for your body temperature to fall. Nor is a full stomach to be taken lightly. As author Debra Gordon graphically put it, trying to sleep on a full stomach is like trying to sleep on a bed of nails. One couple in their early sixties I spoke to literally solved their sleep problems by eating their main meal at lunchtime instead of in the evening.

If you really want to promote good sleep, become what is fashionably known as a 'grazer' and aim for little and often, rather than one or two big meals. Little and often will keep your metabolic rate steady. Remember, also, there are no brownie points in masochism. When you go out for a meal, be a bit kinder to yourself: choose lighter dishes, and skip the pudding. Most of all, *don't* skip meals. To feed your sleep, you need to feed yourself – it's what and how that count.

Good and bad calories

There are two types of calories in the world: empty ones and nutritious, fulfilling ones. Your body will gobble up both, but one sort will nourish it and the other will not. A good calorie is one that comes from real food, its calorific value enhanced by the fact that the food will also contain other nutrients, be it protein, vitamins, minerals, etc., which work synergistically with each other; if it's straight carbohydrate, it's a complex one that takes time to digest, and therefore provides a controlled release of energy. A bad calorie is an empty calorie. All it does is give you a quick shot of energy, so fast it destabilizes your system – leading, eventually, to diabetes.

This is another way of saying that refined foods – in particular white sugar and white flour, and hence the breads, biscuits, noodles, pastries, etc. that are made from them, are not good news. This is not to say you should only eat brown rice and wholemeal bread and never have another fizzy drink. But certainly the less junk food you eat, the better for you, and for your sleep.

Bedtime binges

If you are hungry and haven't had a large meal during the day, accepted wisdom is to have some soothing slow-release carbohydrates in the evening: porridge oats (an age-old sleep aid, as they are rich in both complex carbo and tryptophan, making them probably the most ideal sleep food of all), muesli, jacket potatoes and bananas are all favoured. After eating, a hormone called cholecystokinin is released in the bloodstream, which has a direct effect on the brain, making you feel sleepy and satisfied. The rule is small amounts of easily digested foods. I did the bowl of porridge thing before bedtime for a while; distinctly Winnie the Pooh-like and very comforting.

Bedtime gruel

This is good. Instead of hot milk, soak a level tablespoon of medium or fine organic oatmeal in organic milk for an hour or so in a small saucepan. Then add about a large glass-full of milk and bring to the boil gently, stirring all the time, for a couple of minutes until slightly thickened. Pour back into the glass, add plenty of fresh grated nutmeg, and get into bed. I eat mine with a spoon.

Be nice to your liver

The liver is the largest organ in the body by far, weighing in at around 1.5 kg, and is nature's detoxifier, responsible for eliminating toxins. A scary thought, but as nutritionist Patrick Holford points out, the brain's neurons can't protect themselves from toxins; they rely on the liver to do so for them. It is an immensely busy and active organ, responsible for a staggering 500 functions in total. It converts glucose into glycogen; makes certain essential proteins and carbohydrates if necessary; produces bile, which emulsifies fats, and plays a major role in their digestion; manufactures vitamin A and cholesterol; and stores glycogen, vitamins A and D, many B vitamins, iron and copper. If you want to sleep well, and be well, you don't mess about with your liver. A sluggish liver will affect your whole well-being (hence the term 'liverish'), and your emotional state will affect your liver. Traditional Chinese Medicine teaches that the flow of *chi* (life-force) depends on a healthy liver, that anxiety and depression are associated with liver imbalance, and that a stagnant liver results in fermentation and heat, which causes the body's fire to rise, resulting in poor sleep, anger, agitation and headaches.

Your liver never stops working. If you feed it late at night, it will be in overdrive at 3 a.m. Foods which overload the liver are the usual

zzzz

suspects: fatty foods, alcohol and sugar. The best way to be nice to your liver is to avoid excess, drink plenty of water and take milk thistle (*Silybum marianum*), which both protects and helps to regenerate this vital organ.

Think about your adrenals

If you're stressed, your adrenal glands will also need nurturing. They need a lot of vitamin C (they consume about 90 per cent of what you take in), a constant supply of B vitamins, vitamin D, calcium and magnesium, and omega-3 fatty acids.

Milk and melatonin

Milk products containing extra melatonin are appearing in the shops; they are popular in Finland. In the UK, Slumber Bedtime is an organic milk brand which has four times the normal amount of melatonin, achieved by milking the cows at night. Drinking it will not cure your insomnia but, as they say, every little helps …

Sleep-promoting salads, juices and smoothies

These have been devised by Living Nutrition expert and proprietor of Penhros Organic Hotel and Green Cuisine, Daphne Lambert.

Salads
- Carrots and sprouted wheat salad with tahini dressing
- Wholewheat pasta and pesto
- Hummus with celery and carrots and sprouted wheat bread
- Mixed salad leaves with green peppers, avocado and tofu dressing

Smoothies
- Soaked dried apricots, orange juice, mango flesh and tofu
- Banana, almond milk, tahini

- Wheatgrass juice, avocado, celery
- Blackcurrant, tofu, banana

Juices
- Mango and orange
- Carrot, celery, lettuce, basil
- Cucumber, green pepper, dill
- Wheatgrass, cucumber, celery, lettuce

Sleep supplements

Changing your diet to maximize sleep-promoting nutrition clears away the crud and lays the foundation for better sleep. But it is not a cure. First, nutrients don't work in isolation, but synergistically. As far as sleep is concerned, two obvious examples are the relationship between magnesium and calcium, and that between tryptophan and carbohydrate. The science of nutrition is littered with such examples, and you could drive yourself mad trying to compose the theoretical 'ideal' diet – and it still wouldn't work. Similarly, we all absorb some nutrients better than others (I have the perfect diet, and lousy absorption), need more of this or that than the next person – and we are highly unlikely to be aware of what our precise needs are. I have no idea, for example, of how much vitamin C my personal bio-system thrives on. I just whack it in (as it's water-soluble, excess is just flushed out). All scientists and experts can do is generalize.

This is where supplements come in. They are *not* a substitute for a good diet and sound nutrition, but are potentially a good way of boosting whichever nutrient or sleep-promoting substance you *might* need, which *might* help do the trick.

American studies using magnesium and B complex supplementation, for example, have all resulted in improved sleep for their insomniac guinea–pigs.

Sleep-promoting supplements fall into two broad groups: those which aim to get to the root of the biochemical problem and boost your serotonin or melatonin levels, and those which help you to

z Z z z

relax – and therefore hopefully stop those stress hormones from doing their worst.

Don't use supplements as a quick-fix for not eating good sleep foods; you will need these to make sure you give your body the best chance of maximizing their absorption and doing their bit. They are additions and enhancements, not an excuse for passing the buck.

Nor are supplements cheap. We all experiment with them, with mixed results. I, too, thought GABA was going to be the cure. The promotional blurb is usually backed up by scientific studies, which adds to the hope and usually gives you the excuse you need to fork out. If you are serious about supplements for sleep, you should consult a specialist nutritionist or naturopath who will help determine the right dose for you, and which other supplements you may need. See the Directory (page 266) for addresses.

The more you begin to understand biochemical processes and just how complex they are, the more it becomes obvious (at least to me, and I speak as one who has tried most) why a supplement may or may not work for you. Each of us is a unique, constantly changing, forever interactive mass – or mess – of chemical reactions and electrochemical vibrations. Biochemically, the reason for your insomnia will always be slightly different from the next person's, so your body's reaction to adding anything into the soup will be unique as well. It will also change with time.

Think of supplements as first aid. Remember, too, that unless your insomnia is straightforward – that is, there are no underlying emotional/psychological/life-sorting issues – though proper supplementation can definitely help and does indeed fix many people's insomnia, they are not a magic solution.

Because supplements are manufactured, this raises the question of whether they act in the body in the same way as the nutrients produced naturally. Scientists who frown on their use point to this, though will happily accept sleeping pills and other man-made chemical drugs. Naturopath Tom Greenfield points out that they will be identical to those found in the body, but that the route of entry and the dosage will be different. The decision is yours.

The best and most thorough general account of using supplements for sleep I have found comes from American nutri-therapist and mood-food expert, Dr Julia Ross MA, who runs her own clinic, Recovery Systems, in San Francisco (see www.moodcure.com). Many of the recommendations included here come from her book and are based on her professional experience of treating many hundreds of patients. I must stress, however, as she does, that you should seek expert advice before embarking on a supplement regime, and especially before taking hormonal mood-enhancing or sleep supplements.

For suppliers of all supplements, see pages 254–7.

Supplement know-how

If you want supplements to work, you need to give them the best chance you can. A lot of money could be saved and hopes not dashed by following the basic supplement protocol:

1. The time you take sleep supplements, especially substances like tryptophan, serotonin and melatonin, can be critical. This can often be the reason why such supplements do not seem to be working.
2. You may need less or more than the recommended dose; everyone is different, as is each person's absorption rate. Monitor your progress, and change the dose accordingly.
3. Start with the smallest dose recommended and gradually increase as necessary. Be aware of any side-effects, positive and otherwise. If a supplement really doesn't suit you, stop taking it.
4. Be systematic: try and resist the urge to have a portfolio of supplements unless you know they are going to complement each other and work in tandem, or have been advised to do so by someone who knows what they're talking about.
5. Be *absolutely* sure that the supplement you are intending to take is not contra-indicated with any other medication you may be taking – for example, anti-depressants. Read the labels thoroughly. See also the cautions on page 137.

6. Amino acids should not be taken under certain circumstances, including pregnancy. Before embarking on serotonin, tryptophan or melatonin supplements, see page 137 and take professional advice.

7. Mega-doses of anything can be harmful, so never go mad or take large doses of anything unless under guidance from a qualified nutritionist. See page 266 for details.

How long do I need supplements for?

There is no hard-and-fast answer to this, but generally speaking if you've got the dose right, you should feel the benefits quite quickly, within a week or two. For some it literally works instantly.

With serious sleep supplements, once you've finished the course, stop taking them. Hopefully the imbalance will have been corrected and your body will be topped up. If symptoms return, take some more. Nutritional supplements generally can be taken for as long as you feel you want to.

Serotonin and 5-HTP (5-hydroxytryptophan)

Before it converts to serotonin, tryptophan firsts converts to 5-HTP (5-hydroxytryptophan). This is the recognized way of supplementing with serotonin, and is widely available in capsule form. It is extracted from the seeds of a West African plant, *Griffonia simplicifolia*. All medically-qualified doctors can prescribe it, though not many do. It is found in many of the same foods as tryptophan, but in minute quantities (too little to have a therapeutic benefit). Dr Julia Ross uses 5-HTP supplementation for mood and sleep problems with great success, calling it 'the almost instant solution to low-serotonin problems'. An American supplier boasts it as being the 'biochemical equivalent of a trip to Hawaii'. It has been found to be as effective as Prozac, for example, in relieving anxiety and depression, but without the side-effects.

For sleep, Dr Ross recommends 50–150 mg at bedtime, starting with a single 50-mg capsule. Take another if you don't get to sleep within 15 minutes, and another during the night if you wake up. If you have mood problems (and who hasn't with insomnia?), she says you may need to take 1–3 capsules in the mid-afternoon. Most of her clients need between 4 and 6 capsules per day; larger or more depleted people need more. Use for two weeks.

As Dr Ross points out, serotonin doesn't work for everyone – it didn't for me – especially if your thyroid is not functioning well. It can also cause sleeplessness, vivid dreams, and queasiness in some people. The Nutri Centre (page 254), which supplies it and an information leaflet, suggests not taking it every night, saying that 2–3 times a week may be sufficient.

Tryptophan

Tryptophan is available in pill form as L- tryptophan. It is not easy to find, and cannot be bought over the counter in the UK, though is available on prescription as Optimax. It needs sufficient vitamin B_6, vitamin D and magnesium to convert to serotonin. See page 257 for suppliers.

As a sleep-inducer, it is recommended that you initially take 250 mg about $1^1/2$ hours before bed, plus B complex formula and a calcium/magnesium supplement. Unlike tryptophan taken as food, L-tryptophan is a concentrated form, and converts to serotonin much more quickly. It should therefore be taken between meals, and with no other protein to compete with it. It can raise serotonin levels by up to 200 per cent. Both it and 5-HTP have been found to raise levels of melatonin by over 300 per cent very quickly – in as little as 10 minutes.

The use of L-tryptophan as a dietary supplement is not without controversy – in 1989 a faulty batch produced by a Japanese firm caused 40 deaths in the US, leading to the FDA (Food and Drug Administration) calling for a voluntary ban. Before then it was one of the most widely used supplements in the world, having been clinically proven to relieve insomnia and depression. It was withdrawn until 1995 in America, where it has now been reinstated, and has continued to be used in Europe with no recorded problems. For more about this, read 'The Tryptophan Scandal' in the features section of www.patrickholford.com.

$z\,z_{z}{}^{z}$

Large doses of tryptophan – up to 1,000–3,000 mg – are said to be highly effective for insomnia, but should *only* be taken as a short-term measure and under professional guidance.

Melatonin

The use of melatonin supplements is frowned on in the UK; it is only available on prescription generally from specialist sleep consultants. It is, however, widely used in the US and elsewhere, especially for jet-lag. You can buy it on the Internet, through personal health/well-being mail-order companies (details page 255).

Melatonin won't give you the mood benefits of serotonin, so unless you are a happy insomniac, you should probably try 5-HTP first.

Melatonin supplements are available in tablets, capsules and creams. Tablets and capsules are intended for short-term use only. Take for one week, then stop to see whether you still need it, or can take less. Some experts advise taking it every other day, as it can inhibit natural production. Dr Ross recommends the smallest dose (0.5 mg) at bedtime, by 9.30 p.m., to start with.

It should also be said that using melatonin supplementation is not straightforward and confusion reigns as to when to take it: some experts insist that it needs to be taken during the day, others at night, anything from 30 minutes to 2 hours before going to bed. Part of the confusion seems to be the difference between taking melatonin to reset your body clock to alleviate jet-lag (commonly taken during the day) or using it to help sort your insomnia (usually taken at night). Ditto dosage. It seems that when it works, it can be effective whether taken during the day or evening and in doses ranging from 0.5–10 mg.

Different dosages work for different people, so you have to find what works for you. It is a recognized medical fact that the dose/response range for melatonin is higher than for most other supplements. If you don't respond to low doses (1–2 mg) you are more likely to respond to higher ones (5–10 mg).

I tried melatonin sleep creams for two years without any success. It is, however, a well-established remedy for alleviating jet-lag. Still up for it? Don't try it if you're already depressed, as it may exacerbate your depression. If you find yourself groggy the next day (a common side-effect), try taking it earlier and reducing the dosage. Too much can lead to nausea, dizziness, diarrhoea, constipation, headaches, depression and nightmares.

Children, pregnant women and nursing mothers should not take melatonin; nor should it be taken with anti-depressants or immune-suppressing drugs. It can cause rebound insomnia in some people, so taper it off gradually.

The other way to increase your melatonin levels is to use bright light therapy (see page 194).

Want to know more? Check out www.smartlifenews.com

The case against melatonin

Though there are exceptions, most sleep scientists are generally anti-melatonin supplementation. It's classed as food rather than a drug in the US, and therefore does not come under the same scrutiny that other drugs do. Most sleep scientists claim it simply hasn't been tested enough, and that results using melatonin supplementation are not conclusive. Melatonin supporters do not agree.

Stress-reducing supplements

These work to calm you, make you feel less anxious and generally brighter, and thus hopefully help you to sleep better. Even if your sleep doesn't improve, they can be a very good way of helping you achieve that first important step: getting off the wheel of anxiety. For help with sleep, there are three main candidates.

St John's Wort (Hypericum performatum)

St John's Wort is an excellent anti-depressant. In the UK, the *British Medical Journal* has given this supplement its blessing and has stated it is as effective as any drug for mild depression. In Germany it's the treatment of choice, used far more than conventionl drugs to treat depression. As I know from personal experience and the experience of many other people I have talked to, it works. It also, significantly, boosts serotonin and melatonin levels. Dr Julia Ross recommends it as a backup should serotonin not work. It's available as pills or tincture (tincture is best). For sleep, try taking 300–600

z z z z

mg in the evening, at bedtime, but no later than 9.30 pm. If you need more, take another 300 mg during the afternoon.

As it happens, St John's Wort didn't improve my sleep, but makes up part of the best 'happy formula' I have found to date: St John's Wort and Stabilium (see page 134). So happy, in fact, that for once I didn't worry about my lack of sleep.

St John's Wort can increase your photosensitivity, which means you may sunburn more easily, so be aware of this. As it is an MAO-inhibitor, it may not be suitable for people with blood group O, who have naturally low levels of MAO.

GABA

GABA (gamma-amino-butyric acid) is 'the brain's peacemaker', a stress-busting neurotransmitter which acts as a relaxant and mood-enhancer by instantly neutralizing stress chemicals such as adrenaline; the tranquillizer Valium mimics its action. Biochemically it's an inhibitory neurotransmitter, which means it turns off excitorary brain chemicals and thus calms you down. It's also an amino acid, and supplementing it can help to promote normal amino acid levels in the brain. For some people, taking GABA solves their sleeplessness if it is driven by anxiety. It can be taken on its own or with 5-HTP, tryptophan or melatonin. Dr Ross recommends a dose of 100 mg per day initially. (Patrick Holford suggests 500–1,000 mg).

Too much GABA can have the reverse effect and make you feel more agitated; it also lowers blood pressure – not necessarily a good thing if your blood pressure is low to start with.

Taurine is another amino acid with similar properties to GABA, and is a natural GABA-promoter. Like GABA, it is used to alleviate anxiety and insomnia. The suggested dose is 500–1,000 mg per day.

Rhodiola *(Rhodiola rosea)*

Sold under the American brand name Relora™, this anti-anxiety herbal supplement, also known as Golden or Artic Root, is made from extract of magnolia. It's being hailed as the replacement for Kava-kava, and being promoted as the king of stress-busters. It has been used in Russia and Asia for centuries, valued for its disease-prevention. Like its famous sister ginseng, it's an adaptagenic herb (see below) – one that helps the body correct imbalances, cope with stress better, and restore itself to optimum functioning. It protects and stimulates the immune system, and stimulates fat metabolism (so is also being sold as an aid to weight-loss). It is considered especially beneficial for people who are fragile or easily overstimulated. Trials have shown that Rhodiola reduces cortisol levels and improves the passage of tryptophan and 5-HTP through the brain barrier, resulting in better serotonin levels. Studies have also shown that it reduces cortisol levels and elevates serotonin levels by up to 30 per cent. In trials it helped 70 per cent of participants sleep better, though again didn't do it for me. The recommended dose is 250 mg three times a day.

Adaptogenic herbs

The Chinese have known about these for centuries. Discovered and researched by Russian biologists in the 1950s, adaptogens are plant substances that regulate and normalize body processes and systems, helping them to function in the way they were designed. As such, they often have a wide spectrum of healing properties. They specifically boost the body's coping mechanisms by balancing stress hormones, and thus are especially beneficial for stress. They boost the immune system and also help to diffuse emotional stress and in recovery from physical stress, including lack of sleep.

So far, 15 herbs have been found to be adaptogens, including American and Siberian ginseng and astralagus root.

A note on Kava-kava

Probably the best-known tried-and-tested herbal supplement for relieving anxiety and depression (it has been used in the South Pacific for 3,000 years), Kava-kava was alas banned in the UK by the FSA (Food Standards Agency) in 2003, after claims in Germany that it caused liver toxity. My informant tells me that these were present in the low-quality bark shavings used instead of the root, which is the traditional part of the herb used. No one disputes the efficacy of this natural mood-enhancer – scientists have discovered its active ingredient, kavalactones, which are natural muscle-relaxants and induce a calming effect on mind and body. Like St

z z z z

John's Wort, it works as well or better than prescription drugs, but without the side-effects. It promotes deeper sleep. The suggested dosage is 250 mg an hour before bed. My informant tells me that it's still available in Hawaii. You can also obtain it via the Internet – see page 256.

There are two other herbal supplements commonly recommended to alleviate stress and, therefore, that may help promote more peaceful sleep:

Ashwagandha (Withania somniferum)

Known as the Indian ginseng, ashwagandha, or Winter Cherry, an evergreen shrub, is a much revered herb in Ayurvedic medicine, an Asian aphrodisiac of note and – as its Latin name suggests – is known for its sedative and stress-reducing effects. Another adaptogenic herb, it is said to rejuvenate the nervous system, ease stress and alleviate insomnia. It acts as a sedative, and is widely used in India as a tranquillizer. Most supplement companies will recommend you give it a try. Who wouldn't? Typical dose: 250 mg three times daily. It's my current tincture tipple of choice (along with valerian and wild oats).

Valerian (Valeriana officinalis)

Another one of Nature's Valiums, valerian is well known as a relaxant and aid for better sleep, and is used to treat insomnia as well as stress. It acts on the brain's GABA receptors, enhancing their activity. It doesn't work for everyone – and that includes most insomniacs I know who have tried it – though a recent study showed that although it didn't reduce the time it takes to go to sleep, it reduced the number of times subjects woke in the night, and improved the quality of their sleep. It can be useful for people trying to wean themselves off sleeping pills.

As always, you need a brand with enough therapeutic strength. It should not be taken with alcohol or other sedative drugs. The suggested dosage is 150–300 mg 45 minutes before bed. A bedtime snifter of 30 drops each of Viridian's wild oat (Avena sativa) and valerian tinctures definitely nudges me in the right direction.

What the experts say – natural supplements and insomnia

If there were a magic herbal pill or natural supplement that cured every-one's insomnia, that would indeed be a dream come true. As it is, there are many products which can help enormously. The right dosage taken at the right time and in the right preparation of active ingredient can make all the difference. With Valerian, for example, you either need 150–300 mg 0.8 per cent valerinic acid as the dry powdered extract, or 2–6 ml of tincture, 30–45 minutes before bed.

A good start would be a high-potency multivitamin including B com-plex, antioxidants including vitamin C (to support adrenal function) and essential fatty acids, especially omega-3s (low levels of these are linked to anxiety) – such as organic flax seed oil. In severe cases it's advisable to consult a nutritionist/herbalist to assess other factors, especially adrenal stress – adrenal exhaustion usually causes sleep-/wake-cycle disturbance. Elevated lactate levels are often overlooked, but are another anxiety trigger.

If long-term stress is a factor, you'll need a programme for adrenal recovery – for example liquorice, vitamin B5, rhodiola and vitamin C.

For temporary insomnia or disturbed sleep I would advise an oat-based breakfast, a high-protein diet with lots of magnesium-rich green vegetables, organic juices with carrot, celery and apples, a carbo snack before bedtime, and valerian plus St John's Wort for menopausal condi-tions or for those with nervousness.

For chronic insomnia I would look at endocrine tests (cortisol, DHEA, melatonin) first, then a more personalized supplement profile can be implemented using 5-HTP, rhodiola, etc. When using 5-HTP, it's important to include co-factors such as B_6, niacin and magnesium. Passionflower reduces its breakdown, so is useful to take as well.

— Alex Kirchin, nutritionist and technical manager, Viridian Nutrition

Soporific herbal supplements

In addition to those discussed above, the following herbs are well-known soporifics. Herbal sleep preparations are often sold as blended formulations. I agree with sleep scientists that, generally, lovely though they are, these rarely do the job, especially for serious insomnia. This doesn't mean you shouldn't try them, particularly if your insomnia is recent, temporary, or not that severe. There are countless testimonials from people who swear by them, and for whom they have really helped. As with the herbal anti-stress remedies above, it is extremely rare to experience any negative side-effects. They may not cure your insomnia, but they will not harm you. Use certified organic herbs if you can. Two remarkable American websites that will give you pharmacological chapter and verse about herbs are: www.herbs.org and www.herbmed.org.

German chamomile (Matricaria recutita): So mild and lovely, it is often suggested for children. Add a few drops of the oil to your bath to relieve fraught nerves.

Hops (Humulus lupus): Used for centuries and probably the best known herbal sleeping pill, its sedative effect works directly on the central nervous system. The suggested dose is 200 mg per day; and is said to be most effective taken in combination with valerian, kava-kava or passionflower

Lavender (Lavandular): Who doesn't drown their pillows with it, religiously add it to every bath, or dab the insides of their wrists or soles of their feet with lavender when we go to bed? Aromatherapists swear by its ability to relax you and promote sleep. That includes adding a few drops of lavender oil to children's baths, too.

Passionflower (Passiflora incarnata): This has a proven non-addictive mild sedative effect, and is an ancient remedy in its native South America to combat insomnia. It encourages deep, restful sleep. The suggested dose is 100-200 mg per day, best used in combination with other relaxant herbs.

Skullcap (Scutellaria lateriflora): American skullcap. Used to alleviate anxiety, depression, headaches and insomnia.

See also pages 167 (Flower Power) and 161 (Aromatherapy).

Vitamin and mineral supplements

These are straightforward: your healthfood shop should be able to give you the advice you need. Respected nutritional supplement companies (see page 254) generally operate excellent customer advice services by qualified nutritionists. Just about every book I've consulted recommends you include a multivitamin and -mineral supplement.

z z z z

Calcium and Magnesium

The two most important calming minerals. There are various combinations, but the general advice is you need twice as much calcium as magnesium.

Zinc

Zinc is necessary for mental and emotional health, for the smooth functioning of the blood-brain barrier, and to produce serotonin. It also promotes dream sleep. Buy chelated zinc – it is more easily absorbed.

B complex vitamins

Also essential. There are many brands. You need ones with B_6 and B_{12}. For what they do, see page 113.

Vitamin D

Not called the sunshine vitamin for nothing.

Sex hormones

As explained earlier in this book, low oestrogen and progesterone levels can affect your sleep patterns. For women experiencing the menopause, HRT or its natural equivalents (soy products, progesterone creams, Chinese herbs such as black cohosh) can help raise levels of these hormones (and cure your hot flushes). Though they didn't work for my sleep, they do work for some.

Stabilium

A find. Stabilium is the trade name for garum, the world's first health supplement, and an age-old food supplement-cum-elixir developed by Neolithic man, which food historians will readily recognize as the ubiquitous Roman seasoning you find in ancient Latin recipe books. It's produced in Brittany by salting and fermenting the fish bladders of the remarkable Great Blue deep-sea fish *Garum Armoricum,* which has evolved a specialized physiology to survive in an extremely stressful environment where other fish cannot. As a result, its bladder is a very potent source of antioxidants and neuropeptides, similar to those found in human nerve cells.

z z z z

Stabilium's benefits include relieving anxiety, improving mood, mental alertness, energy and vitality, and enhancing strength. It was given to Roman soldiers, and soldiers in the First World War, and is very popular on the Continent but is not known in the UK. I stumbled across it by chance. Clinical studies in France have shown that it can improve sleep quality, and a three-month study in Japan showed that the alpha brain waves of participants had tripled. I'm a fan. A month's course contains 60 capsules; take it with 3 tablets of St John's Wort a day, and make yourself very, very happy. Available from The Nutri Centre (page 254).

Oats (Avena sativa)

The humble oat is becoming a born-again wonder food. This ancient herbal remedy for anxiety, nervous exhaustion and insomnia is now available in dried and tincture form from Viridian (see page 255). For a recipe for bedtime gruel, and more on oats, see page 119. Organic oatcakes – I like the Nairn brand – come in very handy, too.

Oligotherapy

This will almost certainly be something you haven't heard of unless you live in Switzerland, where *Biologophyt* products, manufactured by the leading Swiss oligotherapy company Laboratoires BioligoSA, are available from health stores and pharmacists. Oligotherapy is the use of essential catalytic trace elements to treat a wide variety of conditions, and has been clinically shown to be especially beneficial for arthritic, immune system and nervous system complaints (which is where insomnia comes in). Biologophyt solutions are said to work at a cellular level, each containing a precisely formulated synergistic combination of trace elements in ionized form for rapid absorption, mixed with plant extracts. The dosage is tiny, just enough to act as a catalyst. If you feel you may be short of trace elements, do try them. They are pleasant to take. The one recommended for insomnia and anxiety is Orange Blossom. To find out more (worth it), take a look at www.bioligo.com (in French and English), or www.oligiotherapy.co.uk. To find a therapist in the UK, see page 281.

What the experts say: nutritional supplementation for sleep

Here are two examples of how to crack your sleep problems using supplements. Please note that both experts stress that the kind of general dietary advice given earlier in this section is also essential. And that you should seek expert help before taking mega-doses of any supplement.

Patrick Holford's Sleep Formula

- Multivitamin and -mineral
- 100 mg vitamin B_6, with 10mg zinc
- 600 mg calcium and 400 mg magnesium
- 2 x 1,000 mg L-tryptophan (if absolutely necessary)

Source: The Optimum Nutrition Bible

Other suggestions from Patrick Holfold, this time from his book *Optimum Nutrition for the Mind*:

- Try 200 mg of 5-HTP with relaxant/soporific herbs for a natural effective sleep-promoter.
- For insomnia specifically, alongside B_6, zinc and calcium and magnesium supplements, 200 mg of 5-HTP, or 2 x 2,000-mg capsules L-tryptophan before bed; herbs such as kava-kava or valerian, or a combination of these herbs and supplements.

Dr Julia Ross's Sleep Formula

The mother of all sleep-supplementation regimes. Please consult the Cautions on page 137 first. For suppliers, see page 255.

- 50–150 mg 5-HTP, or 500–1,500 mg tryptophan at bedtime. If one doesn't work, try the other. You may also need 50–150 mg 5-HTP or 500–1,000 mg tryptophan in the late afternoon to start to build up your tryptophan levels. If neither works, try 300–600 mg St John's Wort mid-afternoon, with another 300–600 mg at bedtime.
- If needed, next try melatonin along with tryptophan or 5-HTP (it sometimes helps to take these every other week). Start with 0.5 mg melatonin, increasing to 10 mg as needed. Take for one week, then stop to see if you still need it; and reduce the dose if you feel groggy in the morning or have any other adverse reactions.
- Be sure to get bright light during the day. If you can't get outside, use a bright indoor light within 1 metre/3 feet of where you are sitting (for more on light therapy, see page 194).

$z^z{}_z{}^z$

- Support with basic supplements: multivitamin/-mineral; 200–400 mg magnesium; 250–500 mg calcium; 1,000 mg vitamin C with bioflavonoids; 400 IUs vitamin D; 10–25 mg B complex; 300 mg fish oil.
- Try 100–500 mg GABA, increase gradually if necessary.
- To relieve stress at bedtime, try the homoeopathic remedy Calmes Forte.

Cautions

For the supplements listed here, Dr Ross offers the following cautions:

- Consult a physician before taking any amino acids, if you have a serious illness (including high or low blood pressure, lupus, migraine, liver impairment, severe kidney damage, an inborn error of amino acid metabolism, an overactive thyroid or ulcers), if you are pregnant or breastfeeding, if you are taking methadone or any medications, especially anti-depressants or MAO inhibitors, or if you have severe mental or emotional problems such as schizophrenia or bipolar disorder.
- If you are already taking serotonin mood-altering medications such as Prozac or an MAO inhibitor for depression, consult your doctor before taking 5-HTP, L-tryptophan or St John's Wort.
- If you have manic-depression (bipolar disorder), do not use St John's Wort or high doses of fish oil, L-tryptophan or 5-HTP without first seeking specialist advice.
- If you have low blood pressure, avoid taking GABA, taurine or niacin, or use cautiously at low doses.

Source: *The Mood Cure*

Exercise

Robbie was a fit young man who played professional football until a horrific car accident left him with dreadful injuries to his face and body, and blinded him overnight. Robbie immediately became a chronic insomniac – he had no sense of day or night, experiencing virtually no sleep, which lasted over a year (90 per cent of blind people experience sleeping difficulties). He cured it by cutting out stimulants, but primarily working out at the gym. Robbie retrained to become a massage therapist, was helped by the Prince's Trust and has been on *This is Your Life*. His story is triumph of will-power over crushing adversity, but also illustrates why every sleep scientist is adamant about exercise and its role in helping restore better sleep.

Exercise keeps you fit and healthy, promotes feel-good endorphins, relieves tension, anxiety and depression, improves well-being and self-esteem, and has a tranquillizing effect. The brain also reacts to exercise by increasing deep or core sleep. Serious exercise can work miracles (see Mike's story, page 139).

To improve your sleep, however, you do not need to go to these extremes. Thirty minutes of moderate-vigorous physical exercise three times a week is, they say, all you need – there are enough studies around to show this is so, especially for older insomniacs who have led sedentary lives and then undertake regular modest exercise.

The important thing is *when* you exercise. Timing is critical. Exercise produces a significant rise in body temperature which lasts for two to four hours and then falls again. Thus, to promote sleep, experts advise exercising in the late afternoon, around 4 to 7 p.m., so your body temperature is falling when you go to bed – which, as we've seen, is a potent trigger for sleep. Conversely, if you exercise too near bedtime, it will keep you awake because your body temperature won't have time to fall again.

In practice, my feeling is it isn't that simple. The 30-minute rule doesn't work for me, but maybe that's because I regularly ran cross-country marathons for 10 years, and my body is used to more serious and lengthy stuff. A five-mile run a couple of times a week didn't improve things either. Robbie works out for at least an hour, as did Mike. Another insomniac friend can only sleep when she works out – but she does this early in the morning before she goes to work. So, though exercise you must – if only for the simple and empowering reason that it will make you feel a whole pile better about yourself – you may need to experiment with what and for how long works for you to send you to sleep.

Any aerobic exercise that warms you up and raises your heart rate slightly above your resting heart rate is fine, including brisk walking, doing yoga, vigorous vacuum-cleaning, digging the garden or walking up stairs. If you want to get a bit more technical, you need to hit your heart rate target zone (see below).

If you currently do no exercise – and lots of insomniacs don't – then you must take it easy, and check with your doctor or a sports specialist first.

When you can't exercise, a hot bath taken one to two hours before bedtime is the next best thing in terms of raising your body temperature so it can fall again in time for bed. And it's bliss. Couch potatoes all cheer now.

Hitting the zone

To calculate the ideal amount of exertion you should aim for when exercising, do the following calculation:

Subtract your age from 220 – this gives you the maximum exercise heart rate – that is, the number of heart beats per minute advisable for you.

Calculate 70 per cent and 60 per cent of this figure – this gives you the upper and lower limits. This is your target zone. To check, rest for a minute and then re-take your pulse, counting the number of heartbeats. Or you can buy a heart monitor wrist device (some gyms provide these) which calculates your target zone and which beeps every time you go above or below this – and won't stop beeping until you're back on track.

Mike's story – exercise works

Mike had suffered manic depression and, as a consequence, insomnia, for over 25 years.

When you are 62 years old, 6 stone overweight, a manic depressive, former alcoholic and ex-heavy smoker, and your doctor says heart trouble and diabetes are looming, there may seem little hope for you. It was my doctor who scared me into action, and through a combination of diet and exercise I managed to lose 6 stone in 18 months. I started to exercise on a very small-wheeled fold-a-way bicycle on which my panting 17 stone 4 lb looked like some circus elephant act. At first I could hardly cycle a hundred yards I was so breathless. I tried each day to cycle just a few yards further. Within a few months I had achieved a self-imposed comfortable, but strenuous, target of six miles – about 25 minutes of cycling – each day. My cholesterol and blood sugar readings dropped to normal and my sleep improved tremendously.

When you have suffered lifelong clinical depression and insomnia, you can imagine how wonderful it is to be free of them, but recovery did not come quickly or easily. The importance of a good diet and exercise was that they empowered my hitherto fruitless attempts to do something about it. It is perhaps strange that something so simple as diet and exercise should have turned out to be the saviour. I commend the process heartily to others who may be despairing depressives (and insomniacs). It's cheap and there are no waiting lists.

Phase Two: Tackling stress

Taking the pressure off

Relieving stress is easier than you think. The trick is to tackle it in bite-sized fashion. As Amanda Geary points out in *The Food and Mood Handbook*, when dealing with stress it's important to understand that everyone reacts to stress differently and has his or her own personal stress threshold.

Take comfort and encouragement from this, too: your body has its own built-in system of checks and balances which enables it to run more or less smoothly – what's known as *homeostasis*. This means we can all cope with a certain amount of stress and imbalance; what we can't cope with is overload.

One thing is medically certain: How we cope with stress is often an indicator of how healthy we are – too much stress will, sooner or later, lead to an increased risk of illness. For this reason alone it's a good idea to make tackling it a priority. Even if you can't do anything about the big stress-drivers in your life, having a tool kit to enable you to take the pressure off the worst of it will significantly increase your well-being and potential for better sleep.

Helen's story – the angry insomniac

Not many insomniacs own up to feelings of anger; we try to be civilized and contain it, turning it inwards, though if the truth be known we often feel irrational anger, especially towards those we share our lives with. Helen, 26 and a media executive, has lived with insomnia all her life, and vocalizes what many who experience regular sleep-deprivation feel.

I sleep very well for 50 per cent of the time; the other 50 per cent I am plagued with insomnia, or what I call 'conscious wakefulness'. My mind won't shut off and I spend the nights in constant conversations with myself, not feeling like I've slept at all. It's a huge issue for me, and going to bed is a nightmare. I try and read myself to sleep, but the anxiety builds up as soon as I close my eyes – that awful 'will I get to sleep tonight?' business. If I don't sleep, I function appallingly. When I sleep, I'm smiley, friendly and optimistic. When I don't, I get angry, especially if it coincides with my periods, I'm pessimistic, lose my enthusiasm, am not pro-active, argue with my boyfriend and can't raise a smile for love or money. My boyfriend sleeps like a log, and that pisses me off, and I get really annoyed with myself for not being able to sleep like he does. In fact, I get furious with my whole body because it won't do what it's supposed to do, yet feel powerless to do anything about it. I also get really angry if I'm woken up or disturbed in the night. It's the worst thing in the world. People just don't understand how fragile sleep is for someone like me and how I don't have the ability to fall back to sleep the same way that they do – so much so that the only 'safe' environment for me is one where I know I can't be disturbed.

I've tried all the herbal remedies but none of them has worked for me, and I hate taking sleeping pills. I'm now at the time of my life where I really want to try and do something to improve my sleep. I went to the doctor and he advised counselling, which I don't want. I know there are probably unresolved issues fuelling my insomnia, in particular job issues I have to face, and other things I need to change in my life. Ironically, considering counselling has brought new anxieties into my life which are bigger than the anxiety over sleep, but because they're tangible, I can do something about them – as a result, the sleep is improving. I've also recently taken up yoga, and find time just before I go to bed to do a few exercises and try and ground myself and chill out. Tackling anger is next on my list.

Assessing your stress levels

This is the first thing to do. Identify which of the factors outlined on page 31 you feel are causing you stress, and reassess each one accordingly. To recap, major stress drivers can be physical (diet, environment, bad sleep hygiene, too much exercise), mental (worry, anxiety, being too obsessive, etc), emotional (family and personal relationships) or spiritual (finding your place in the grand scheme of things).

Dr Max Luscher's Diagnostic Colour Test

If you'd like to try a painless but penetrating analysis of your stress levels, this test can help. It has been in clinical use worldwide for over 50 years. I found it gobsmackingly accurate in my case. The test is cheap, takes 30 seconds to do, and could not be simpler. You are given five coloured cards, each with a number, which you choose, one by one, in order of preference. The results are analysed and your stress level calculated. Just be prepared for a few surprises. For more, see www.luscher-color.com. To see (and do) the test on-line, visit www.actualsystem.com/products/colortest/luscher. Or get in touch with Spring Gardens Clinic (see page 267).

Combating stress to improve your sleep

Here are four simple but profoundly important self-help steps:

Step 1. Be at peace with your insomnia

The stress caused by worrying about the fact that you can't sleep, and coping with its debilitating side-effects which leave you weary, irritable and unable to cope, makes up the vicious circle we all know only too intimately. Number one priority, therefore, is knocking this stress on its head. For more, see page 175.

Step 2. Learn to relax

This is covered on page 146, and really works. The effects are cumulative: the more you learn to relax, the more chilled out and relaxed you become, and the more being relaxed becomes second nature.

Step 3. Remove the sources of stress

It took me three years of chronic insomnia to learn this one, but removing myself from my normal life for a few weeks – for me this meant a cozy cottage in Hereford to begin writing this book – worked wonders. The layers of stress peeled off and my sleep improved, which gave me the confidence to know that I could sleep for 3–4 hours straight without constantly waking up.

It is not a long-term solution, and is often the most difficult aspect of relieving stress to enact, but if stress is caused by work or personal life issues, and this is fuelling your insomnia, physically removing yourself from that source is, I believe, crucial. It allows you to cut the stress chord and gives you precious breathing space, and through this helps you to gain a different perspective.

A cottage did it for me, but there are other options. The key is to keep it simple and minimalist. Having the *holiday* of your life is not the same. You need the *space* of your life. I would argue it should be ordinary and normal, but that's what worked for me. Retreats, for example, have become a popular antidote to the stresses of modern life (Microsoft tycoon Bill Gates, they say, goes on one every year). They suit some people better than others, but are another obvious option. The Retreat Company (www.theretreatcompany.com) is a good place to start, and offer a free help service. If you have the funds, booking yourself into a holistic spa is heaven. Or you could try walking. There is something about reducing your world to the pack on your back and having nothing else for your brain to do except enjoy the scenery, cope with the weather and get to the next night's accommodation that's very restorative. Britain is blessed with several long-distance walks, which can be broken up into manageable stages. It doesn't have to be a marathon and you don't have to do all of the Pennine Way – just the bits you fancy. A canal holiday on a traditional longboat has a similar effect. You can't go very far in a day, or do very much, but it's a journey just the same.

Step 4. Change your thoughts

This is covered in detail on page 176. For relieving stress, however, it's not just a question of changing your thoughts about insomnia, but changing them generally. Cultivate optimism in whatever you

z z z z

do. Even if you aren't an optimist by nature, become one. Have that silver cloud permanently pinned up on your wall. It's as good a medicine as laughter – and there is plenty of scientific evidence to back this up. As I recently read, cheerfulness and good health walk hand in hand. Some therapists advocate setting goals. I'm working on it.

Three simple stress antidotes

Laughter
Laughter is the best antidote to stress. It relaxes you, activates feel-good hormones, boosts the immune system and helps keep you healthy. You don't need jokes or funny stories to make you laugh. Finding humour in your own situation, however dire, and being able to laugh at yourself (and your insomnia, when you can) are all you need. It lightens the load, relieves stress and is one of the easiest and most pleasurable cures at your disposal. And the reason why the cover of this book has a funny cartoon.

Get a pet
My chiropracter keeps nagging me to get a dog. Pets are very healing; they alleviate depression and relieve stress. They need exercising, too. I'm on my way to the pet shelter.

Squeeze it out
This is a stress-reducing exercise devised by Eldon Taylor (see page 228). Your new dog will be able to play with the ball, too.

Get a squeezable, spongy yet firm rubber ball that fits comfortably in your hand. Since stress levels build up unnoticed, make it a practice to squeeze your ball at intervals throughout the day. While you squeeze it, think about letting all stress and tension go. If you know of something that has stressed you, think of it and put the stress into the ball, then just squeeze it out over and over again.

Relax and let go

The ability to relax is something we all need, but insomniacs tend to need it more than most. We are not talking about watching TV, retail therapy, having a night out with the girls or boys or even going for a walk in the countryside, however uplifting that might be. *Deep* relaxation is what we mean here, the kind that reaches your inner core, enabling you to relax, as it were, from the inside out. Such relaxation brings two benefits: it dissipates and neutralizes stress (and therefore the hormonal roller-coaster it triggers), and helps calm brain waves – and a calm brain is much more likely to be a soporific one.

Relaxation also helps to keep you healthy. The science of Psychoimmuniology (PNI), which investigates the relationship between the mind and the immune system, has shown that relaxation techniques strengthen the immune system, which makes you less vulnerable to illness. No surprises, then, that this section just grew and grew.

Deep relaxation is not automatic. You need to learn how to do it, make it part of your life, and practise it every day; the effects are cumulative. I have discovered, too, that you can never have enough. What works for me is to have a kit of different simple ideas and techniques that I can dip into frequently throughout the day. Relaxation music CDs are on most of the time when I'm working, doing household chores or cooking, for example.

Deep relaxation involves one or more of three basic techniques: muscle relaxation, breathing deeply, and being quiet and still or calming the mind. Reading about the latest scientific thinking on relaxation reveals that Eastern philosophies have been right all along: yoga, tai chi and meditation are prime examples of how to relax deeply.

Massage is another option, and La Stone therapy is bliss.

z z z z

What works for me

Two suggestions that have changed my life:

TV, Radio, Newspapers

A few months ago I took a decision not to watch TV, listen to the radio or read newspapers. People I know are aghast, but the results for me have been remarkable. At a stroke this made my life, and me, feel so much more peaceful. I seriously believe every insomniac should try it – it could make a huge difference. After all, it's what most people do on holiday. It also creates space in your life for other thoughts, and enables a more spiritual-like calm to enter your life. You don't need to be a Trappist monk or adopt a code of silence – soothing music is fine. Nor do you need to dump the TV or radio in the tip. Just make it a rule only to watch or listen to your favourite feel-good programmes, read your favourite magazines, and so on.

Washing Away the Day

The standard advice for insomnia is to have a hot bath in the evening. My alternative is to take a warm bath just before bed, light a candle, put on some music or a meditation/insomnia tape, add some aromatherapy bath oil – then sit there in the dark, watching the candle. The water should not be more than comfortably warm. If the weather is hot, have it as cool as you like. In any event, by the time you get out you should feel cool.

Sit there for at least 30 minutes and up to an hour; as long as it takes for you to wash away the day and leave it in the bath-water. It's the best way I've found to clearing your head and putting that symbolic full stop between your day and the night ahead. It also gives you space to be with, and cherish, yourself.

You can also try this sleep mantra: 'Tonight I am going to sleep for X hours.' Choose the number of hours you really want, and repeat several times, talking to each of your major organs, affirming how sleepy they are, especially the left side of your brain. Get the right brain to put the left to bed, and suggest the right side talks to you in your sleep. Your family will think you have gone totally mad, but when you read the section entitled 'Using the Power of Your Mind' you may see why it makes some sort of sense.

Get out, dry yourself gently and pad off to bed, having previously got your bedroom ready. Spray/massage/dab on more essential oils or whatever you do that is part of your nightly soothe-me-into-sleep ritual.

Yoga and Tai Chi

Two great mind-body disciplines. Whether you use them as a means of getting yourself fit and flexible, improving your well-being or for their spiritual dimension matters not. There is nothing bad and everything good about them. New research in the US is looking at the potential benefits of yoga specifically for helping insomniacs to sleep better. The results so far are encouraging.

Yoga

Yoga has become so much part of Western life it needs no introduction. Re your sleep, to have a noticeable effect you are probably going to have to do 30–45 minutes of poses, breathing and meditative techniques that specifically relax you and calm the nervous system. These include the Child's and Cat Pose, and kneeling and seated forward bends. To be of real benefit you will also need to do your practice every day. You should do the postures gently and, ideally, hold each posture for a few minutes (the longer you hold a posture, the better the desired effect). Alternating the Child's Pose and Cat Pose is lovely. The Cat Pose releases tensions from your spine, and the minute you bend over into the Child's Pose you feel like going to sleep.

Breathing techniques should emphasize exhalation, which is about letting go, rather than inhalation, which tends to energize and activate the nervous system (good for the morning, but not at night). Don't try to breathe in hard, and aim to make the exhalation long and lingering. Alternate nostril breathing (see page 149) is specifically recommended for calming the mind.

z z z z

Yoga will certainly help get your body and mind into relaxation mode, but will suit some people more than others. For example, I love my yoga to bits, but until I found viniyoga (see below) I was the kind of person who needed to go to a class rather than struggle on my own. For others, their daily yoga practice is sacrosanct and as much a part of their life as cleaning their teeth.

The kind of yoga you do is also important. Energizing postures are for daytime; in the evening or before you go to bed you need them to be slow and calming. If you are specifically thinking of making yoga part of your better-sleep strategy, I would advise asking a yoga teacher to help devise a specific set of exercises for you. For a specific bedtime meditation, see the Kundalini yoga website, www.kundaliniyoga.org.

Viniyoga

Not as well known as some of the other forms of yoga, but one that may suit you and your insomnia. It has certainly helped me. Its guiding principle is the application of yoga to the individual, and not the individual to yoga. Though some practitioners give classes, and they organize occasional workshops, it is usually taught on a one-to-one basis, each practice or set of postures tailor-made for the client. The precise use of the breath and sound alongside the postures is another defining feature. I think of it as yoga for the 21st century – it's like having a personal trainer, except they don't work on your abs, but on what you need to maintain harmony.

I was initially given a set of three elementary postures that anyone could manage, interspersed with simple breathing, that took 10–15 minutes to do. The practice made me softer, which is exactly what I needed. For more, see www.viniyoga.co.uk.

Alternate nostril breathing

The left hemisphere of the brain is associated with male energy (logical thinking, judging, investigating), and the right with female energy (intuitive thinking, lateral thinking, compassion). Breathing through the left nostril activates the right hemisphere, and vice versa. Our breath naturally regularly changes from one to the other. At any given time, one nostril is dominant and easy to breathe through, whereas the less dominant one feels like it is blocked.

Alternate nostril breathing – blocking off one nostril at a time – is a way of harnessing and balancing these two opposed energies flowing through the nervous system. It is used as a form of meditation and is said to be especially useful for Air (Vata) types, who are also prone to insomnia. The key pre-bedtime is that the air flow must be easy, soft and gentle with no forcing in or out, coupled with a smooth transfer of air from one nostril to the other.

This is the basic version: block off your right nostril using the thumb of your right hand, by pressing it gently into the side of your nostril, alongside the bony bit. Breathe in through your left nostril, then close this off with your third finger and exhale through your right nostril. Breathe in through your right nostril, close it off, and exhale through your left – and so on. I do this before bed. Not authentic, but I like to sink into the exhalation, using the breath as a means of letting go or winding down from the day.

Middle-of-the-night relaxation technique

Having a simple relaxation ritual for the middle of the night is very useful. Everyone agrees that deep breathing is the key. This is just one variation on many; it's easy enough to devise your own. Don't go bull-at-the-gate, though. Nice and easy all the way.

1. Take a quiet, deep, rhythmic breath, using your abdomen (place your hands on your tummy and breathe so that your hands rise with your tummy). Hold the breath for a count of four, then exhale slowly and gently, aiming to expel the air from a place deep down in your groin, feeling yourself relaxing and letting go as you do so. Follow your breath, not your thoughts.

2. Take another deep breath; count to four as before. As you exhale, imagine yourself relaxing from head to toe – think of it as a shower if you like, cascading down, and feel the relief as the relaxation spreads throughout your entire body.

z z z z

> Repeat this as often as you need to, or until you reach your boredom threshold. If you can't manage this, breathe quietly from your abdomen, focusing entirely on the gentle rise and fall of your tummy and the in and out of your breath. You will probably find it sounds and feels like the gentle swell of ocean waves. Very quieting and comforting. Then think of something nice.

Tai Chi

Tai chi is remarkable, and the ultimate art of gentle and profoundly graceful relaxation. I love it. Though if you think standing on one leg being a rooster is easy, think again. Tai chi has its roots in Martial Arts.

Tai chi seeks to establish equilibrium between the two universal energies, *yin* and *yang*, and to increase *chi*, the life-force, and is a proven method of reducing stress and anxiety. It grounds and earths you, and acts specifically on the major energy centres that correspond to the body's main nerve plexes and endocrine glands, which control your bio-rhythms, including the sleep-wake cycle.

Taoism teaches that when muscles tighten due to stress, blood vessels are constricted, thus restricting the flow of *chi*; your mind also has 'virtual' muscles which get stressed when there is a lot on your mind. Tai chi is a system of calming both, allowing *chi* to flow again. The postures are made up of constantly flowing movement. Although different from yoga postures, they, too, exercise all parts of the body, build suppleness and massage the internal organs. Yin postures use soft, round, smooth and flowing; yang postures are the opposite, expressed in hard, angular movements. Often, they involve practice with a partner. Breathing, visualization and meditation are its other main aspects. Practice enables people to release the negative emotions often associated with insomnia, such as fear and anger. This 'clearing out' and ability to reconnect can be an invaluable aid for better sleep.

Like yoga, tai chi is not a quick fix. Though a weekend's course or 10-week taster will give you a good introduction, it takes time to master the postures, and you need a good teacher. You will need to practise, too – ideally every day for at least 10 minutes a day. Angus Clark's *Elements of Tai Chi* is an excellent introduction. He also runs courses internationally – see www.livingmovement.com. If you live in London, the British tai chi champion, Michael Jacques, organizes several courses throughout the city. For more, see www.taichiuk.co.uk.

Chi Kung

The sister discipline to tai chi, this focuses more on individual work, centring and awareness, and on cultivating *chi* to promote well-being. The postures are mostly stationary. I spent a memorable weekend in France, north of Paris, under bright blue skies in freezing temperatures learning the art of being still, under the careful eye of Madame Kar Fung Wu. At the time, running cross-country marathons seemed easy by comparison. No wonder, then, that, as one Martial Arts instructor reminded me, *Kung* means 'hard work'.

Meditation

I have several friends who meditate, including one devotee who, if she can't sleep, will sit up in bed and meditate instead, and who reckons it is as restorative and refreshing as sleep itself. Everyone I know who manages to stick at it, swears by its benefits. Like yoga and tai chi, it is an entirely Good Thing with no detrimental side-effects. Meditation has been proven to encourage slower alpha brain waves, so no wonder people who meditate have a calmer outlook on life; it has also been shown to reduce biological ageing. Latest research shows it can be similar to Stage 1 sleep.

Though we don't stop to think about it much, our daily consciousness is spent in a constant internal dialogue with ourselves. It's exhausting, and in many ways self-limiting. Meditation counters this and reconnects you with your intuition. As one advanced practitioner puts it, it's an uncoupling process which frees the mind from the negative emotional energy attached to the actualities of daily life. Change tension to *attention*, and the tension will go. Experienced meditators also report that it enhances deep sleep, facilitates more efficient dreaming and gives greater clarity to your dreams, enabling you to use that 'dream data' in your waking life.

It doesn't matter which meditative technique you use: all aim for the same place, which is that inner calm and sense of being – the space between the thoughts – leading ultimately to greater awareness, and the ability to access different levels of consciousness and connectedness with the universe. Some techniques use mantras, some chanting, visualizations or your breath. You can meditate with your eyes shut or open, and can spend hours or just a few minutes a day at it.

If you've the mind and temperament for it, meditation is great. For insomniacs, however, it is not necessarily easy. I learned TM (Transcendental Meditation), enjoyed it and was grateful for it, but stopped when insomnia hit hard, simply because I couldn't face sitting with my eyes closed for another 40 minutes a day, when I had spent so much of the night doing precisely that. As one yoga teacher gently pointed out to me, meditation is actually hard work. Keeping the chatter at bay is the universal problem, but asking an insomniac to quiet or 'watch' his or her mind is to misunderstand what we actually spend a good deal of the night engaging in.

This is not to say you shouldn't think seriously about giving meditation a try. I'm now trying eyes-open meditation for short bursts of time, which suits me better. As Dadi Janki, now 87, of the Brahma Kumaris World Spiritual University (www.bkwsu.org) says, one minute every hour can make a tremendous difference. For many people meditation really does improve their sleep. It works (its name comes from the same Latin root as 'medicine', meaning 'to cure'), and can change peoples' lives. Just don't necessarily expect automatic relief (or enlightenment). Purifying the mind, a necessary first step to true or higher meditation, can take a lifetime. Lower your sights, and the discipline of sitting or being still and learning the art of peaceful concentration is an accomplishment not to be sneezed at, which will help deliver the relaxation benefits you need.

Meditation tapes and CDs tend to be a bit New Age-y, which may or may not be your thing. For beginners, I would recommend Richard Lawrence's *Meditation – A Complete Workout for the Mind* DVD/CD/cassette (www.richardlawrence.co.uk), which is refreshingly down to earth. Not music to meditate by, but Bliss CDs (www.blissfulmusic.com) are profoundly meditative, calm and uplifting, and will nudge you (spiritually) in the right direction. For more useful contacts and websites, see The Sleeping Directory (page 235).

What the experts say – sleep, insomnia and karma

As a firm believer in karma (what goes around comes around), I believe there is a good reason for everything, including insomnia. From a spiritual perspective, insomnia for some people is an expression of a higher part of themselves – their spiritual selves or soul – crying out to be listened to, which has probably been neglected in the hurly-burly of life. To use John Lennon's phrase, life is what happens when you are busy making other plans. Not sleeping, in these cases, can be a way of forcing your spiritual or deeper consciousness to the fore – an attempt, if you like, to have its fair share of the action. Sufferers of this kind can be said to have a 'spiritual deficit' – they can be people whose inner nature is particularly spiritual, even though they may not perceive themselves that way, and hence who find themselves troubled when this spirituality is not fully expressed in their daily lives. The remedy is to redress this deficit. Meditation, which connects with your intuition and inner you, is excellent for this.

With insomniacs there can also be a left/right brain imbalance. Most of us spend too much of our time living busy left-brain lifestyles, so that the right hemisphere, which is our creative outlet, becomes starved. Perhaps you need to find a way to express your creativity, for example, through arts, crafts or hobbies, and thus experience the peace that flows from them.

For some people, not sleeping – that is, the inability to reach deep sleep – is a way for the mind to try and engage with those brain wave frequencies that are not being provided for during daily life. The brain has become habitually programmed to the beta state in the daytime, and some of us are subconsciously desperate to experience the alpha and theta states before reaching sleep. We are attempting to experience these before passing into the deep sleep state – and this, ironically, can lead to more beta activity. Again, meditation, which naturally induces the alpha state, would be a remedy for this.

z z z z

Deep breathing – the full yogic breath, using your diaphragm to draw in 'prana' or 'chi' (the life-force) – affects both your waking and sleeping life. The more you can learn to practise deep breathing, the more calm and 'in balance' you will become.

Affirmations and visualization are also tremendously beneficial in combating insomnia; the trick here is to really mean it. If you do that, it works.

– Richard Lawrence, secretary of The Aetherius Society,
author of *The Magic of Healing*

Instant meditation

Yogis will no doubt frown, but even insomniacs are pushed for time. One of the most helpful suggestions I've had is from a video producer who teaches meditation, who first gets her pupils to pause for a moment several times a day. It's like adding punctuation marks to your day, which gives you a momentary pause and works really well. If you don't try any other form of meditation, try building these little full stops into your day. Go inside yourself for a moment, breathe and let out a sigh. Sighs, apparently, are very good for you too.

Progressive muscular relaxation

A well-known method to release tension, this is used by sleep therapists as a tool to help you go to sleep and get back to sleep when you wake up. It costs nothing to learn, and will take about 15–20 minutes to complete. It's usually done lying down (in bed is fine), but can also be performed sitting up. The result is a very warm, tingling and relaxed you. This is how to do it:

Starting with your feet, clench each muscle group in turn until you can feel the muscles are beginning to strain, then relax. The order is: right and left toes and feet, calves, thighs, buttocks, fingers and hands, arms, back, neck and shoulders, face. For example, you do the right foot first, then the left, not both together. Every time you've finished one group, take a couple of deep breaths, noticing the warmth generated.

Because it's active, this is less monotonous than some techniques. You also get to find out pretty quickly where you hold tension. Like all relaxation therapies, you need to give it a fair trial. If, like me, you need props, *Beating Insomnia* (page 290) comes with its own free CD which includes a very good progressive relaxation exercise.

Finally, and not in the least bit progressive, but if you're fidgety in bed (which means, by the way, that your *vata* is rising), tensing yourself – squeezing every muscle you've got, all at once, not forgetting the ones in your face – then letting go, can sometimes do the trick.

Autogenics: 'my right arm is heavy'

Autogenics is the Western answer to Eastern methods of relaxation, emotional balance and inner peace. Sleep scientists recommend it, and it is used in the aviation industry to help air crews correct disturbed sleep patterns. The term means 'generated from within'. It's a life skill for dealing with, among other things, the negative effects of mental and physical stress. The autogenic state of relaxation additionally facilitates re-balancing of the left and right brain hemispheres, and leads to greater emotional balance, a strengthened immune system, etc. Numerous clinical papers attest to its usefulness.

As long as you have the commitment (important, this) and discipline to sit or lie quietly and be able to say a few monotonous phrases to yourself invoking heaviness and warmth – the same feelings, incidentally, that sleep invokes – such as 'My right arm is heavy,' nothing could be easier. As one therapist explains, 'It's a self-help mind and body therapy, which is short, simple, logical and methodical. It has rules and if you follow the rules, it works.'

The key is passivity. With autogenics you aren't going anywhere, trying to achieve or analyse anything. You begin by taking a mental check of your body, then saying the phrases to yourself three times a day, either sitting or lying down. The goal is deep relaxation, achieved by silent passive observation of each part of the body in turn. Its gentle, repetitive nature quickly induces a Pavlovian reaction of switching to the resting state of body and mind, a kind of surrendering to the moment (as with repeating a mantra, repetition switches off the body's stress response). A session when you go to bed is actively encouraged, as the autogenic state nudges consciousness towards sleep.

The relaxation aspect of autogenics is immediately appealing, but it's the positive affirmations – 'I am at peace' – that I like for bedtime. These simple devices for dealing with life's tensions and negative emotions are very powerful. The exercises are soothing and soporific, but also monotonous. People with a low boredom threshold, like me, take note: there will be times when you will struggle. To find out more, and before you invest in that purple yoga mat, take a look at www.autogenic-therapy.co.uk, which includes a list of UK practitioners. Courses last 8–10 weeks.

What the experts say – autogenics and insomnia

Autogenics is particularly suited to deal with sleeping problems and insomnia. Most clients who are not sleeping well enjoy better sleep very quickly, usually within 2–3 weeks. Their dreams may become more vivid and the quality of their sleep improves as the deep relaxation kicks in. We may then introduce a supplementary technique, known as intentional offloading exercises, to deal with the underlying causes. Clients do this in private – it's a simple, safe way of speaking or writing out your emotional baggage in order to shed it. One client described it as 'self-psychotherapy'. During this process their sleep may temporarily be disrupted. This is common with any holistic therapy and is the cathartic effect of the body–mind system regulating itself back to normality. Sometimes the opposite happens and clients return reporting they've slept for 10 hours every night and still feel tired; this usually lasts a very short time and is the forerunner of some real improvements. In my sleep workshops I also emphasize sleep hygiene and obvious lifestyle changes such as cutting down caffeine and good night-time routine. I work with clients individually to see what changes would fit into their lifestyle and are likely to make a positive difference to their sleep patterns.

Insomnia is rarely a single-cause complaint, and everyone needs a different solution. Autogenics is fundamentally a self-regulating technique to enable you to help and heal yourself. As therapists, we are there to guide you to your own solution, we show you the way through and leave

z z z z

you to do it yourself. This training works well in the majority of cases.

— Christine Pinch, autogenic therapist and
co-author of *Autogenic Therapy*

Hypnotherapy tapes

These can really work. Indeed, hypnosis is recognized as the fastest way to induce deep relaxation. For anyone who struggles with muscle relaxation techniques, I thoroughly recommend it. The trick is finding tapes that work for you. I was lucky. For me, Pilgrim Tapes (page 253), in particular their stress-release, rapid relaxation and insomnia tapes, have been very beneficial, but I have listened to others that leave me cold. For more on hypnotherapy, see page 225. See also InnerTalk™ CDs, page 228.

Massage

Massage is the most popular relaxation therapy. It encompasses a variety of techniques, traditional and new. I know one sleep scientist, for example, who favours Japanese Shiatsu massage for insomnia (it uses specific sleep-promoting acupressure points, and for some people really does the trick). I have one friend who has three different sorts a week, and swears they keep him healthy.

Unless you use massage as a form of pampering yourself, most of us feel that being pummelled is part of getting our money's worth. Aiming for the neck and shoulders, which is where most of us (myself included) collect tension seems common sense, too. For insomnia, however, naturopathic practitioner Stewart Mitchell, author of *The Complete Illustrated Guide to Massage*, explains that this may be exactly what some of us *don't* need:

> When we can't 'drop off' to sleep, there is too strong a demand for blood in the head (which accompanies worried thinking) and less circulation deep into the core of the body, which ensures sleep.
>
> Although your head may feel rough enough in the daytime to want it massaged, it would be better, if you are having disturbed sleep, to have treatment which draws pressures downwards. In particular, slow deep

treatment of the arms and legs, and superficial trailing strokes to the trunk reduce stimulation to the head. For chronic insomnia, the emphasis should be more on the legs.

How long before you will feel some improvement depends on stress levels, but you should aim for a couple of massages within 10 days, then at weekly intervals for up to six weeks. If you have the opportunity to sleep for a little while after the massage, all the better.

Massage is immensely intimate, and building up a relationship of trust with your massage therapist is important. (If you don't feel comfortable being touched or stroked, better to try acupuncture instead – see page 220.) As another leading massage expert and best-selling author, Clare Maxwell-Hudson (www.cmhmassage.co.uk) says that once this trust and feeling of safety have been established, it is possible to massage someone to sleep. I agree. To promote sleep she recommends an early evening massage and the use of sedative, calming essential oils. She also says what calms you suits you best, be it stroking your face or feet. The easy solution? Buy your partner a massage book and essential oils, and get them (and yourself) booked into an introductory massage course. Clare Maxwell-Hudson's *The Complete Book of Massage* covers everything, including reflexology and a Shiatsu treatment for insomnia.

Massaging babies

Another tip from Clare. Getting babies to sleep can be a nightmare in itself. Research has been done which shows that when you rock a baby, he or she will indeed often fall asleep in your arms – but will wake up again when he or she is put down. Gently massaging a baby produces the opposite effect. The baby is alert while having the massage but, when put down, falls asleep more quickly. Again, combine the massage with aromatherapy. *Aromatherapy and Massage for Mother and Baby*, by Allison England, is an excellent starting place.

The Shiatsu mattress

This could be the answer to your massage dreams: Shiatsu massage by remote control, in the form of a portable Japanese acu-massage

z z z z

table. Switch on and the padded ergonomic rollers or 'fingers' embedded in it roll up and down your neck, spine and legs, in a wave-like manner, stimulating 44 Tsubo energy centres. People who have used it rave about it for reducing stress, aches and pains, headaches, lethargy, tiredness, sports injuries and more serious complaints such as fibromyalgia. It boosts circulation and aids detoxification. In the UK you can trial it first, or hire it from Back in Action shops, or raid the bank and buy one (current cost around £2,400). It will certainly pinpoint trouble spots: these will hurt, sometimes acutely, but in time the sore points melt away. By the time I found this my relaxation regime was clearly working, and my body lapped it up. I experienced hardly any touchy points at all. If you know you are tensed up, however, this has to be worth a trial. For details, see page 253.

Neck and spine stretchers

These simple wooden stretchers have cushioned rollers that you lie on, cradling your neck and spine. Developed by back specialist Neil Summers, they relieve tension in the two areas where it collects most. Though lying on smooth knobbly wooden rollers doesn't feel like it, they gently massage and stretch the vertebrae, relieve disc pressure (thus alleviating back pain) and ease and remove mechanical muscular tension that accumulates along your spine, giving you the equivalent of a deep Shiatsu massage. The neck stretcher is also recommended for easing headaches. You use them for a few minutes each day – immediately before going to bed is a good idea. The result is a more relaxed, less anxious you. I have a neck stretcher, which definitely releases tension in my neck. Available via mail order, online from www.thebackcoach.com, or from Back in Action shops (page 253).

The magic pillow

Don't raise your hopes too high. This is a small circular wooden bowl with four pressure pads that cradles the occiput bone at the base of your head. It was invented by a cranial-sacral and physiotherapist, Ged Codd. Technically it's a 'still-point' facilitator and eases tension. It can help alleviate anxiety, depression and

z z z z

fatigue, and promotes better sleep (and better digestion). You only need to use it for a few minutes a day, and you can use it in bed, too. Available from the inventor direct (page 251) or at www.thebackcoach.com.

Getting the fire out of your head

Something you will come across often, for example in chat forums or on radio chat lines, and which I use frequently in the small hours when frustration is setting in, is simple hydrotherapy. How well it works depends, I find, on your anxiety/alert levels. You have nothing to lose by trying. This is my version.

When you can't sleep, go to the bathroom and place your wrists under running cold water for 60 seconds. Do this until they feel very cold. Rinse your face, arms, neck and shoulders with cold water, too. Shake off the excess. Return to bed. The idea, again, is to cool you down and reduce the flow of blood from your head, helping it to switch off.

Aromatherapy

Aromatherapy has been around since before Biblical times, and is one therapy which has come of age. Even the NHS now use lavender in some hospitals to promote sleep. Though aromatherapy is highly unlikely to cure your insomnia, as one aromatherapist friend reminded me, the sense of smell is a powerful relaxation tool. For this reason alone, the use of essential oils can be very effective as part of your wind-down process at the end of the day. Their therapeutic benefits in relieving stress-related conditions is well known; indeed, oils noted for their relaxing properties such as clary sage, frankincense, lavender, sandalwood, sweet marjoram and ylang ylang have been shown to stimulate serotonin production.

Essential oils work directly on the autonomic nervous system. Applied to the skin, they enter the bloodstream; inhaled, their scent has a direct effect on mood centres in the brain (which is why most aromatherapists believe inhalation has more effect). Combining

z z z z

aromatherapy with massage – a marriage made in heaven – is acknowledged to be the best and most efficient way to reap benefits. I am a convert; these days my bedroom and bathroom are choc-a-bloc with essential oil products. Adding them to your evening bath or night-time massage, is perfect. The effect continues afterwards, so it's recommended you give yourself an hour or so before you go to bed (I don't bother). Combining essential oils with relaxation techniques, especially deep breathing, or using them to self-massage (experts recommend the soles of your feet, which helps release tension collected during the day) is perfect, too.

Aromatherapy primarily addresses the emotions. A consultation with an experienced aromatherapist, who will take a case history and devise a blend of oils uniquely for you (smell each one first to see if it suits you – that is, if you like it – a small but important tip) and specific to your insomnia and its perceived causes, is to be recommended. Ideally, choose someone who is also an experienced masseur.

The second option is DIY. There are a bewildering number of products out there to try – drops, lotions, 'remedy rolls', 'pillow mists', candles and such like. Except for serious bath oils, I remain to be convinced about most of them. Pillow mists, for example, sound fine, but the ones I have tried stain your pillow cases. Be aware, too, that high-quality essential oils do not come cheap. Like all natural remedies, if the concentration is not sufficiently strong to be of therapeutic benefit, or the oils are poor quality, they won't work. Look for the words 'pure essential oil' on the label. Aromatherapy is also a skilled art. For all these reasons, blended formulas by respected brands are your best bet. Aromatherapy Associates (www.aromatherapyassociates.com), for example, supply leading spas worldwide. Their gorgeous Deep Relax bath oil does just that, and remains the one that works best for me. The irresistible Comfort & Joy (www.comfortandjoy.co.uk), who produce bespoke oils and excellent bath and face products, are another find. Other quality brands that have developed specific 'sleep easy' or 'deep relax' products include Aroma Therapeutics™, Dreamline™, Elemis, Quinessence and Origins. Materia Aromatica specialize in essential oils from organic and wild plants, and Allison England in aromatherapy products for pregnancy, new mums and babies. For details, see page 259.

Finally, as I have discovered, aromatherapy is not just pretty-smelling essences. To learn more, start with www.quinessence.com (excellent on-line shop as well) or, for an industry perspective, www.a-t-c.org.uk. Aromatherapy aficionados will like www.fragrant.demon.co.uk, which includes a global search for aromatherapy suppliers and practitioners.

Which essential oils to use?

Speak to people in the business and they all come up with slightly different hit lists. This is the definitive one.

Bergamot (*Citrus bergamia*)	Refreshing, uplifting.
Benzoin (*Styrax benzoin*)	Soothing, warming, comforting, sedative. Recommended for insomnia caused by worry. Note: Some people may be sensitive to this oil.
Clary sage (*Salvia sclarea*)	Deeply relaxing, warming, anti-depressant; imparts feeling of well-being. Recommended for stress and depression. Note: heightens the effect of alcohol; do not drink alcohol when using this, as it may also produce vivid dreams (presuming you get to sleep, that is).
Frankincense (*Boswellia carteri*)	Alleviates fear. Balancing, relaxing meditation oil, noted for its rejuvenating skin properties.
Jasmine (*Jasminum officinalis*)	Despite its fabulous fragrance, a 'male' oil, strong and confidence-building. Can be one of the best to promote sleep, but also one of the most expensive. If you like it, it quickly becomes addictive. Recommended for insomnia, apathy, and nervous exhaustion.

z z z z

Juniper (*Juniperus communis*)	Detoxifying, relaxing.
Lavender (*Lavendula officinalis*)	Best-known and most-used essential oil for sleep. Commonly recommended for insomnia, but also an all-purpose oil. If you've used it a lot, though, take a break and try something else.
Melissa (*Melissa officinalis*)	Alleviates grief; fortifying, strengthening, uplifting. Recommended for insomnia, shock, anxiety.
Neroli (*Citrus aurantium amara*)	Relieves anxiety; uplifting, restorative, relaxing. Commonly recommended for insomnia.
Petitgrain (*Citrus aurantium amara*)	Balances nerves, relieves irritability, promotes sleep.
Roman chamomile (*Anthemis nobilis*)	Soothing, relaxing, calming, and good for headaches. Forget chamomile tea, this has a rich, warm fragrance. Often recommended for insomnia.
Rose (*Rosa damascena/centifolia*)	Quintessential 'female' oil – nurturing, comforting, relaxing, good for your skin; especially recommended for grief. Also recommended for insomnia and nervous tension.
Sandalwood (*Santalum album*)	Must be genuine high-quality Indian or Australian sandalwood. Grounding, calming meditation oil. Recommended for insomnia, depression and nervous tension.
Sweet marjoram (*Originum marjorana*)	Relaxing, especially good for aching muscles, sedative. Recommended for insomnia, anxiety and nervous tension.
Tangerine/mandarin (*Citrus reticulata*)	Soothes the nervous system; recommended for tense people who can't sleep.
Valerian (*Valeriana officinalis*)	Uplifting; currently undergoing clinical trials in Germany to calm hyperactive

z z z z

children. Well known to alleviate insomnia, though not often used as its aroma is strong and unpleasant. Said also to improve sleep quality, and to leave you more refreshed when you wake up.

Vanilla (*Vanilla fragrans*) Calms and softens anger, frustration and irritability. Maybe we need to eat more real vanilla ice-cream?

Vetiver (*Vetiveria zizanioides*) Noted for its relaxing effect on the nervous system.

Ylang ylang (*Cananga adorata genuina*) Grounding, relaxing, anti-depressant. Recommended for insomnia, nervous tension, stress and excitability.

Aromatherapy burners

A silent electric crock vaporizer is best, and safer than those that use candles to warm the oil. This kind also allow whichever blend you're using to do its stuff through the night. Worth the investment if you are going to get serious about aromatherapy. Don't forget to check how much hum other kinds of electric vapourizers make if you are considering them. For where to buy one, see page 259.

Aromatherapy candles

The candles are lovely; the wicks generally frustrating, such that I've never managed to buy one that lasts more than halfway down the candle.

Elemis soothing lavender eye pillow

A soft eye mask filled with lavender and flax seeds, which surprisingly is wonderfully comforting and has become my latest must-have. You place it on your closed eyes (it doesn't have a strap) and use it to relax before you go to bed (though I also use mine *in* bed). Soothes tired or upset eyes, and good to take travelling. Readily available. For more, visit www.elemis.com.

z z z z

Aromatherapy face creams

I don't care what anyone says, your face and skin are what suffer – and show most – when you don't sleep. Aromatherapy night creams do two jobs in one. Night-A-Mins by Origins (part of the Estée Lauder group) is not that expensive and I think very good (I also like their petite 'Resume the position'™ diffuser, which comes in a handy cartridge that you keep under your pillow, and use when you wake up.) Comfort & Joy's Facial Soother moisturizing oil could be just what your skin needs, too. Frankincense, neroli, rose otto and fennel are the ones to use on your wrinkles.

Aromatherapy: Top tips

Passed to me by Marie-Louise Carey-Morgan, a skilled aromatherapist and masseur. Remember, too, that different essential oils work synergistically together.

1. Pure essential oils are very potent. Less is more. In a bath, use 6–10 drops.
2. Always add essential oils when the bath is full; this allows the globules to disperse properly. To make sure, swish the water around.
3. Change your blends, or essential oil(s) frequently. Your body gets used to the same essential oil(s), and their effect wears off in time (true).
4. Respect essential oils. They are powerful chemicals and their effect can be very strong. Except for lavender or tea tree oil, do not apply pure essential oils directly to the skin. Some may have occasional side-effects – for example, citrus and melissa can cause skin irritations.
5. Store somewhere cool and dark, out of direct sunlight.

Flower power

The use of flower essences, be it in aromatherapy or as remedies in their own right, as discussed here, is one of the most gentle and pleasant methods for promoting calm and relaxation, and alleviating emotional difficulties. It is difficult not to find them appealing: everyone loves flowers. That they work is not in question; the degree with which they will help you sleep better is. Personally, I think of them as support and nourishment.

The power of plants to heal (phytomedicine) is an expanding discipline, and there are several companies worldwide who offer plant essences made from liquid tinctures. All capture the healing life-force of the plant, using the energy of sunlight to transfer and 'imprint' the active component into distilled water. For the best account of what they are and what they can do for you, read Richard Gerber's *Vibrational Medicine for the 21st Century*.

Phytobiophysics flower formulas

These use the vibrational energy of plants to heal. There are 20 master flower formulas, created from thousands of different essences, formulated as tiny pilules. Their creator, Dame Diana Mossop, explains that they act as neurotransmitters, instantly regulating the system being targeted and redressing energy imbalances at all levels.

For insomnia, you need Flower formula 4, thistle. It acts on the brain and central nervous system, and balances the circadian rhythm. Benefit will take anything from 1–3 weeks. They are available by mail-order (page 259) and can be taken with homoeopathic remedies (many homoeopaths use them) as long as they are taken 15 minutes apart.

The term 'phytobiophysics' describes a complete diagnostic and holistic healing system, of which the flower formulas are just one aspect. The method of analysis employed is referred to as The Heart Lock theory, which assesses the primary area of weakness and isolates 'tissue memories' responsible for your present physical and emotional malaise. Four types of tissue memory are traced: physical, mental, emotional and spiritual. Diagnosis also reveals your heart type (a similar concept to that of Ayurvedic *doshas*), which shapes your constitutional blueprint, plus any specific nutritional deficiencies.

You can either see a qualified therapist (see Directory) or have a postal consultation with Dame Mossop at her Institute of Phytobiophysics in Jersey: you simply send a saliva sample for

z z z z

analysis (swabbing your mouth with a cotton bud will do). You receive a written diagnosis and personalized prescription in return. Mine was spot on: flower remedies 2 (recovery), 4 (tranquillity) and 9 (appetite), an energy-harmonizer to counteract a polio vaccination, and nutritional supplements co-enzyme Q10, choline/inositol and glutamine. It took a couple of weeks, but I and my sleep became more tranquil. Current cost is around £65 for the consultation, plus remedies. For more, visit www.phytobiophysics.com.

Bach flower remedies

These are truly lovely: very good for the soul, hit and miss for your insomnia. They alleviate emotional maladies and, like homoeopathic remedies, work at the vibrational level and aim to change negative emotions into positive ones. Many practitioners swear by them. White Chestnut is the remedy specifically recommended for sleeplessness, being overwhelmed by persistent thoughts that go round and around your head, and when you are a prisoner of your thoughts.

Often a mixture of various remedies will be recommended, or you can make up your own prescription that will most closely match your mood and feelings. For example, early on in my insomnia I was advised: olive (exhaustion), pine (guilt), Star of Bethlehem (trauma) and Wild Oat (purposelessness) as well as White Chestnut. Make of that what you will. Ainsworths (www.ainsworths.com), who remain faithful to the original Dr Edward Bach method, is the brand usually recommended, and the ones I use.

For American, Australian and Amazon Forest flower essence companies, see page 259.

Music and sound

Using music to help you relax is one of the easiest ways to de-stress. Music feeds your brain as well as your emotional well-being. Mozart's music, for example, has been shown to resonate at deeper levels of consciousness; the sound of a crystal or Tibetan bowl, when struck, will fill your whole being. Relaxing music and sounds can also lower brain waves and heart rate (listening to Albinoni's *Adagio* is one of the most famous examples of this phenomenon). A nice thing to know, too, is that if a piece of music seems relaxing to you, it is. For me, for example, it's Gregorian chant.

Don't forget that the opposite is also true. Wailing dolphins may be music to some people's ears, but will leave others wondering what all the fuss is about.

Today there is a whole industry devoted to soothing relaxing music specifically to help promote sleep. Until I developed insomnia I would never have thought of using them. Now, I'm a convert. Playing them before you go to bed, and in bed, can also make you feel safe and secure. So much so that silence during the night now seems uncomfortably quiet. Just remember you need a CD player which switches off silently, or has a repeat button. Another tip is to play the music softly: the aim is to create a soothing environment, not recreate the Albert Hall. Go to a specialist shop, ask your friends, get recommendations from therapists and, if possible, borrow them first. Hitting the spot takes effort, and can cost you plenty if you get it wrong.

For some people, certain voices or radio programmes have the same calming effect as music – Radio Test Cricket coverage is one well-known example. Many people who have difficulty sleeping sleep with their radio permanently on, burbling away softly in the background. I have one insomniac friend who plays story tapes in the small hours. Hypnosis tapes quickly become reliable dummies as well.

Scientists and music are merging fast. Spanish geneticists have recently produced a CD tape of 'DNA music'; maybe a serotonin and melatonin adagio is the miracle cure we need.

Symbiosis

Symbiosis (see below) are a remarkable trio who compose much-lauded music specifically for use by complementary practitioners, which has been proven to reduce heartbeat rate. Their music has an experimental and experiential quality to it – think New Age plus serious musicians; ironically, it engages your attention and I find is best listened to, say, in the bath, when you can indeed let your mind float freely. They are meant to be played softly. They have a free 24-hour music line (020 8781 0755) which means you can get a taste first. Very restful but don't expect 'wallpaper', New Age or otherwise. For details, see page 264 or visit their website at www.symbiosis-music.com.

What the experts say – music to sleep by ...

Your body naturally responds to rhythms: the slower the beat and the less discernible the rhythm, the more your heartbeat and brainwaves will slow down. Indeed, when composing music to seriously calm you, it's the 'space between the notes' and timbre of the sounds rather than the melody, tune or rhythm that matter most. Ideally, music for relaxation should create an internal space that the listener can literally step into and float freely with, discovering their inner peace. Music played only on synthesizers doesn't work as well as that which includes real instruments, because only these allow the notes to breathe. Gongs, bells and Tibetan bowls are often used for their healing effect, but if not sufficiently muted can sometimes have hard angular notes which can 'awaken' you. What you need is soft, rounded sounds. Flutes, acoustic guitar, oboe, cor anglais and the cello are perfect examples. Ideally, too, you don't want any emotional involvement with the music, or be familiar with the tune. This explains why the gentle ebb and flow of the ocean is nature's ultimate 'sleep-by' sound to help you drift off.

– Clive Williamson, musician and producer with Symbiosis

Sound therapy

Music and sound go beyond relaxation, so much so that using sounds and tones to relax and rebalance your own vibrations is a 'becoming' therapy. Although as ancient as time itself, sound therapy is at the distinctly New Age end of the therapy spectrum, though there's real science to back it up. For example, sounds naturally fall into two groups: deep, gentle relaxing tones such as 'ahhh', or stimulating notes such as 'eee'. As far as improving sleep, relaxing tones encourage brain waves to become slower; the alpha–theta border, at around 8 Hz, is thought to be the optimum healing frequency. You can also use rhythm such as drumbeats to train the heartrate to beat slower, a practice Native Americans have used for centuries.

z z z z

Sound therapists use sound to detect and correct imbalances and blockages, and aim to get clients into the magic 8-Hz state. Lyz Cooper of Soundworks, who runs her own Academy of Sound Therapy, describes sound therapy as re-tuning body, mind and spirit, and believes that sound, as she puts it, dislodges things that have been hanging around on a physical and emotional level. She offers the following simple relaxation/stress-busting suggestion, suitable for anyone who sleeps solo or has a partner who sleeps so deeply nothing will wake them. For their CDs see page 264.

> Breathe gently and deeply with your hand on your tummy, which should rise and fall. As you exhale, say 'ahhh', softly and gently, like a sigh. Repeat several times. Using the sound 'ahhh' relaxes the body and gives the brain something to do, distracting it from the chatter. Use this when you are in bed, or when you wake up in the night.

Colour therapy

Blue is the colour you need: blue skies, blue oceans, blue anything. It's a 'cooling' colour. Richard Gerber in *Vibrational Medicine for the 21st Century* states that recent photo-biology research has confirmed that blue light has a calming effect on the nervous system. It is also considered to be the primary colour of the throat chakra. Computer healthscan programmes usually include a colour analysis. Mine? Blue, of course.

Insomnia tapes and CDs often include suggestions on using the colour blue, and invite you, for example, to visualize yourself being wrapped or enveloped in a soft blue mist, or breathing blue into your body, penetrating you completely right down to every cell. Which I also do occasionally, usually in the bath.

Magnets as sleep aids

The medical use of magnets to treat illness, alleviate pain and arthritis, heal sports injuries faster, boost the immune system and energy levels, enhance blood and lymphatic circulation and aid in detoxification – and help you sleep better – is well established in Russia, China and Japan, and is fast gaining credibility in the West.

Though there have been many clinical trials and progress being made, no one is yet really sure why bio-magnetic therapy works. It is generally agreed that the therapeutic use of magnets simulates the earth's magnetic field, creating the optimum conditions for the body to self-heal. Everyone also agrees that they are neither magic nor a miracle cure. Nor are they a new idea: magnetic substances have been used to heal for over 2,000 years.

About 70 per cent of people who use magnets find them beneficial. For enhanced results, some practitioners advocate their use alongside other healing therapies.

Their use is not without controversy. Some experts frown at the thought of mucking about with your own electromagnetic field, and point to the need for more research on the effects of fixed magnets. Then again, you could take encouragement from the fact that modern magnetic therapy was first developed through space exploration (astronauts wear suits lined with magnetic materials to stop them from being ill). For the definitive (and very, very long) account of bio-magnetic therapy, take a look at www.healthplusweb.com, key in 'biomagnetic therapy' and check out *Biomagnetic Healing* by Gary Null.

Magnet pillow pads and mattresses

Type 'magnet therapy' or 'bio-magnetics' into your search engine and you will be confronted with an array of American companies selling magnet aids. The ones that light up for insomniacs, or anyone who wants to sleep better, are pillow and mattress pads. In Japan, apparently, one in three people sleep on them; in one trial, over 75 per cent of patients reported significantly improved sleep, and 15 per cent of insomniacs likewise. Susan Clark, in *What Really Works*, says that researchers have found that sleeping on them balances acupressure points within 15 minutes, and that the longer you sleep on them, the faster the body rebalances itself in this way.

Norstar (page 253) supply high-quality, high-strength pillow and mattress pads (thin quilts in which small magnets are embedded). Drinking lots of water to flush out the toxins released during their

z z z z

use is mandatory. Norstar also advise drinking North Pole magnetized water – achieved by placing one of their magnetic coasters under your glass. This is said to facilitate communication of the electromagnetic force between cells.

Many insomniacs report huge success using them. I found the pillow pad, recommended in non-severe cases, was not as comfortable as the mattress pad, which you place under your sheet. This was one cure I really wanted to work. Who knows? That it didn't do anything for me may just mean that magnetic aids are hit and miss for something as complicated as insomnia; as one doctor commented, they address your symptoms but not necessarily all the causes lurking in the deep recesses. But you can at least try them for a month, and if they don't help, send them back and get a refund. Not that I did – the lure of all the other potential benefits was simply too great a temptation; plus Norstar's magnetic Neo discs sorted out my painful shoulder in a trice.

Magnetic aids should *not* be used by everyone – if you have a heart condition, pacemaker or are pregnant, seek advice first.

Using the power of your mind

Pick up any self-help book on curing insomnia, and the central key will be changing your behaviour patterns and attitudes towards your insomnia. This is borne out by every insomniac I have talked to who has managed to create some sort of equilibrium. I know this to be true from personal experience, too – being chilled out about your insomnia dramatically improves the restful quality of your 'nonsleep'. This is what I call 'power relaxation', and is the one behavioural adaptation that has been key for me.

It's also borne out by clinical studies. The book *Seven Days to a Perfect Night's Sleep* cites a recent two-year study where most of the participants who used behavioural therapies no longer qualified as insomniacs, whereas half of those who took drugs still had insomnia.

The behavioural and attitude changes you need to make are all simple, straightforward and predictable. But they do take discipline. Changing every negative thought about last night's awful struggle sounds fine in theory, but often falls short in practice. You can only pretend so much, only dig deep so far. There are times when you feel truly miserable, and telling yourself it was fine really doesn't cut the mustard at all. Just try to remember that getting angry with yourself because you're supposed to be positive and can't manage it today only sets up another layer of anxiety. Being perfect or exacting your own miracle cure is not what it's about. It's about making a concerted effort to do the best you can. This will, I promise, yield results.

Bill's story – Been there, done that

Bill, 28, has had insomnia for as long as he can remember – his earliest memories are of not being able to sleep. He has learned to live with his insomnia, is used to operating perfectly well on very little sleep, and has found his own way of managing it.

> Since I was very young I've had trouble sleeping; for me, it's specifically the process of actually drifting off to sleep itself. One unfortunate fact is that I'm almost always only able to sleep at night and in a bed; I can't have afternoon naps, or fall asleep on trains or planes.
>
> The remedies I've tried have included variations in room temperature (both higher and lower), natural sleeping tablets, other herbal applications, different pillows and mattresses, and the timing of exercise and also of dinner. I don't drink tea or coffee, so this has never been a factor. I have to say that, of all the herbal treatments (and, to a lesser extent, pharmaceuticals) that I've tried over the years, none has worked in the slightest. Even being particularly tired, physically or mentally, doesn't guarantee sleep. State of mind doesn't seem to be a factor either, as it can happen when I'm completely relaxed mentally. I've found I just sleep best when most comfortable, including a good pillow and an empty bladder!
>
> On a very, very good night I'll get 6–7 hours' sleep – but this isn't normal; I've got accustomed over the years to 3–5. The major insomnia kicks in when I fail to sleep at all; these patches can last up to a week, but normally last 3 or 4 nights. Over the years I've developed a back-up for when this happens. I've become able to simply stay relaxed and in bed; I wouldn't call it meditation, but perhaps something akin to that. For me, it's the next best thing to sleep. This way the body gets rest even if the

mind doesn't; even keeping my eyes closed helps reduce bags and eye ache. I don't panic the way I used to when I couldn't sleep; I just get on with it and avoid getting up or fidgeting or worrying. Again, having a comfy bed and pillow helps a lot here.

Mind power

No scientist today would deny the body–mind connection or the awesome potential of that cognitive part of us that we can't see, feel or touch, but with which we engage every second of our lives; or that the mind is the most powerful healing force we have at our disposal. The power of the mind is so great that people can literally grow younger and make miraculous recoveries from serious illness or accidents. It is the power of the mind, conscious and subconscious, that enables simple changes in thoughts and behaviours to have desired physical effects, and which is at the heart of so-called cognitive restructuring techniques to solve insomnia.

'I think therefore I am' is not philosophy but fact. Body and mind talk to each other constantly; and every thought produces a predictable physical or chemical response in the body. As Marisa Peer puts it in her book, *Forever Young*, beliefs create biology. Science is proving this fast: biofeedback techniques conclusively prove that altering mental activity has a direct effect on your autonomic nervous system. As we each have around 60,000 thoughts a day, each having some micro- or macro-effect on our body chemistry, it is easy to see how we become victims of our thoughts and become a bundle of habits – not sleeping well being one spectacular example.

Equally, you can change your mindset and belief patterns by consciously changing your thoughts; this in turn has a corresponding effect on your body chemistry. Put crudely, positive thoughts release positive chemicals that support the immune system (the immune system and nervous system are inextricably linked), whereas negative thoughts and emotions mobilize the stress response and release chemicals that have deleterious effects. Negative thoughts also prime the brain's wakefulness system and weakens its sleep system. It's as simple as that.

For example, if you think of yourself as old, you will indeed age more quickly. A famous experiment in 1979, conducted by Dr Ellen Langer, a psychologist at Harvard Medical School and author of the book, *Mindfulness*, took a group of men over 75 years old to a retreat for seven days where everything had been changed to mirror 20 years' previously, and in which they had to act and be as if it were 1959. Their age, as determined by a range of bio-markers from muscle mass and hearing to blood pressure and hormonal output, was measured before and after. After just seven days of living as if they were 20 years' younger, all the patients had reversed their biological ages by 7–10 years. Nothing else had changed: they didn't take more exercise, live on organic juices, play hypnosis tapes or fall in love.

Less ambitious examples are equally revealing. A recent study by Professor Gruzlier, a neurophysiologist at Imperial College in London, found that students who visualized white cells fighting off viruses and bacteria suffered significantly fewer infections than the non-visualizers.

It's the same with insomnia, which is why hypnotherapists and doctors like Dr Greg D Jacobs, author of *Say Good Night to Insomnia* who has spent 10 years at Harvard Medical School researching and treating insomnia, have so much success with many of their patients.

The caveat, of course, is that it doesn't work for everyone. Some people are naturally more self-motivated, some prefer medication, and some find themselves better suited to sleep-restriction therapies. The point, however, is that believing in mind power is an enormous resource, no matter which road to recovery you decide on.

Negative to positive

If we all felt positive about ourselves and our lives all of the time, we wouldn't need doctors and we wouldn't get insomnia half as often as we do. Nor would a whole multimillion-dollar motivational industry have grown up to convince people that they have the power to fulfil their own potential and create the lives they want.

Therapists who use mind power point out that the mind cannot hold two conflicting views at the same time. To take an obvious

z z z z

example, there's no point saying to yourself 'I can sleep' if that small voice inside you is saying the opposite. The knack is to replace or modify negative thoughts with plausible positive thoughts, ones that *do* make sense and ring true, that you *can* believe in; in other words, to put a positive spin on whatever negative thought passes through your mind about your sleep, and to see the cup of insomnia as permanently half-full rather than perennially half-empty. The mantras at the end of this section (page 184) are very good examples of these kinds of positive thoughts. You then bolster this up with reinforcing statements such as 'I know I can sleep' and 'I will sleep'. If you say them often enough *with conviction*, they will eventually sink in.

This is because your subconscious doesn't have the capacity to judge (Deepak Chopra once said you can trust your gut feeling better than your brain, because your gut cells haven't yet evolved to the stage where they doubt what they think), but presumes if you do something often enough you want it that way. Once your subconscious accepts the idea, it remains firmly lodged until another idea dislodges it. The longer a negative thought is implanted, the more difficult it is to budge. This is why tackling negative beliefs about your insomnia are best dealt with as soon as possible, before they become too entrenched in your subconscious.

If this kind of thing doesn't come naturally to you (and it doesn't with me), it will sound a bit hollow at first, and you will probably feel a bit of a fool. The more you persevere, however, the easier and more natural it becomes. It is also surprising how quickly you can begin to feel more relaxed about your sleep and not let the insomnia dominate you as much as in the past.

The hard bit initially is banishing all negative thoughts; every time you catch yourself, whether silently or out loud, you have to replace that thought with something more positive (and you probably clock up many more than you think; my average is about 20 per day). This takes discipline, but again, practice makes perfect – or as near as imperfect non-sleepers can manage.

Write it down

Writing down your negative thoughts and changing them into positive ones makes them real; and a real thought will become a real belief faster. This is why all books which aim to harness mind–power have exercises where you write everything down, generally in two columns, side by side, so you can see the difference. This is where language comes into its own. A slight shift in the kind of word you use can make a tremendous difference to the intent of the phrase. Apart from minimizing negative words and accentuating positive ones, there's no fixed script. The point is to find the words and phrases that press the right bells for you. For a few examples, see page 179.

Being realistic

Part of the problem with insomnia is that we tend to want too much, and our goals are set too high. We all dream and wish for

8 hours' sleep every night, despite the fact that this is the exception rather than the rule for most normal sleepers – or, as already discussed, that most of us get more sleep than we think some or most of the time. Lowering your expectations to be more realistic, and equally not distorting things out of all proportion, are essential first steps and will impinge directly on your success with changing what Dr Greg D Jacobs calls the NSTs (Negative Sleep Thoughts) into PSTs (Positive Sleep Thoughts). In other words, give yourself a break, and don't make it any more difficult for yourself than you need to.

For articles by Dr Greg D Jacobs, visit: www.talkaboutsleep.com.

For more on Cognitive Behavioural Therapy, see page 198.

Positive insomnia

These are examples of how to turn negative and dreary thoughts about your insomnia into positive, more palatable ones.

Negative thought	When I wake up, I can't get back to sleep.
Positive spin	I'll fall back to sleep sooner or later, when my body is ready.
Negative thought	I can't get enough sleep.
Positive spin	I don't need as much sleep as I think. I can function very well on less.
Negative thought	I feel dreadful today/can't do a thing.
Positive spin	I don't feel that bad; If I take it easy and only do what I feel like doing, I'll be fine.
Negative thought	I'm at my wits' end, I've been awake most of the night.
Positive spin	This has happened before, and I know that I'll get through. I don't need to be a star every day.

When all else fails, and you can't sleep, try this one:
'Sod it. I don't care.' (It can be amazingly liberating.)

Or (sneaky, this):
'Sleep is my best friend. It blots things out.'

Or (where you need to be):
'I give myself permission to sleep.'
'Sleep is safe and serene.'
'Sleep gives me a second shot at my life.'

If you use insomnia cassette tapes or CDs, say to yourself:
'Great. I don't have the responsibility of getting to sleep. That's [name of person/tape you're listening to]'s job. He/she can get me to sleep and I'll just daydream ...'

'Every day in every way ...'

Affirmations – willing yourself better – are all part of the mind game and have definite healing benefits. The original, and still one of the best was developed by Emile Coué, a French pharmacist a hundred years ago. Think of it as a mantra (which, essentially, is what affirmations are):

Every day, in every way, I am getting better, and better, and better, and better, adding for good measure *and my sleep is becoming more peaceful.* Say it three times – with feeling. Repeat often.

Power relaxation

Power relaxation is not a method but an attitude. It's a determination, first, to seek out relaxation therapies that work for you – be it something simple like listening to your breathing when you lie in bed awake or needing to work out every night in the gym – and secondly to train yourself to be still and calm during the night. It's 'positive resignation' if you like, but it works. To achieve this, all you need to do is to use three simple techniques, in whichever combination suits you best:

z z z z

a) a method to relax the body
b) visualization
c) banishing negative thoughts and being kind to yourself by thinking of comforting positive statements instead of fretting and worrying.

Visualization

Visualization – using your imagination – is bread and butter for the subconscious mind, just like facts are to the cognitive brain. As such it is an extremely powerful therapeutic tool – used extensively, for example, in hypnosis, psychotherapy, meditation and relaxation techniques, and, increasingly, to help patients overcome serious illness.

Though fundamentally only an extension of day-dreaming, which we all do, it is not something that comes naturally to everyone. Only two-thirds of us are classed as visualizers – say 'banana', they see a banana, not the word. The rest of us are not. We have a sense of banana and maybe what it tastes like, but we don't automatically see one.

Visualization techniques are used frequently by a variety of therapists to help combat insomnia, and appear regularly in self-help books. As a non-visualizer I find them of limited usefulness, but for many people they really work well. It is also a fact that if you do start using visualization techniques, either to help relax or to lull yourself into positive sleep mode, you will quickly improve your ability to visualize.

Two simple and well-known ones that I have used and find useful are:

Sleeping visual

See yourself tucked up in bed fast asleep. You may want to see yourself at a time when you did sleep well – in childhood, for example. Be sure to put yourself into a really cozy, comfortable bed, with soft comfy pillows, your best blankets, that the bedroom is decorated and furnished exactly how you want, and is in a safe environment or a place where you feel happy and contented.

z z z z

Worry filing cabinet/box/balloon visual

This is for putting your worries, cares and anxieties away last thing at night. Choose whichever carrier appeals most.

1. Put your worries neatly into a file(s), close the file(s) firmly, and file them away into a filing cabinet. Lock the cabinet and walk away.
2. Put your worries in a box. Visualize the box – its colour (mine is polka-dot yellow), how big it is, etc. You can turn your worries into little creatures and put them gently in the box and put them to bed, use real people – whatever suits. Shut the box tight and put it somewhere safe for the morning.
3. Put your worries into a hot air balloon. Again, visualize the colour of the balloon and set it in some gorgeous scenery with blue skies and fluffy white clouds. Undo the ties and let your cares, worries and anxieties float away. This one gives you and your worries a holiday.

Blocking it out

You can't think straight in the middle of the night, and can't resolve problems, big or small. We all know, too, that things look different in the morning, and whatever you agonized over in the middle of the night is usually irrelevant, or you change your mind, or something. Training yourself to understand this, and to banish automatically and religiously whatever worry is on your mind, simply by saying to yourself 'It'll sort itself' or 'I can't do anything about it now, I'll see things more clearly tomorrow', is extremely valuable. The aim is not to deny the problem, but to be pragmatic. In short, think about nice things in bed, however fantastical they may be, and keep the day's row with the boss, or tomorrow's exam, for the morning.

Michael's story – The thinking insomniac

Michael, 60, a professional psychotherapist, is in a better position than most to understand what's happening with this thing called not sleeping.

z z z z

Insomnia fascinates me. I have a keen interest in all aspects of the subject, and read everything I can about it. My parents were terrible sleepers and resorted to pills. Some of my clients suffer from it, too. It's the demon *par excellence* that cuts you down to size and prevents you from being at your best, or fully living.

I've suffered from insomnia for 20 years. On a good night I'll get 5–6 hours; on a bad one, 0–2 hours. There's no obvious pattern; the slightest thing can trigger it off, though Sunday night, before returning to work, is probably the worst night. Just the passing thought on Sunday evening that I might not sleep that night is enough to prevent me from sleeping. It's like the flick of a switch. The nights I am most likely to sleep well precede days when nothing out of the ordinary, be it pleasant or possibly unpleasant, is likely to happen.

I've coped with my insomnia by sensitive psychological management and meditation, so that even if I don't sleep I remain peaceful. I learned early on that getting anxious about not being able to drop off made things worse. I have a second bed downstairs, which I resort to for a fresh start and to avoid disturbing my wife's sleep. I've dubbed this 'the sleep factory'!

I've learned to live with it, but there's no doubting the difference normal sleep makes. Although I wake feeling more groggy than usual and more reluctant to get up, I soon begin to feel that I have more depth and substance, and delight in feeling lively right through the day.

It's not difficult to formulate a psychological explanation which may account for my own insomnia demon. What is being undermined is a 'compensatory drive' to live life to the full, to be fully present. Many of us are driven to want more and be better, striving for something like the perfect life (and the perfect sleep to sustain it). In subtle ways this may engender self-controlling processes which can run counter to the simple surrender of control needed to fall asleep. When I'm lying awake, I sometimes think of TS Eliot's powerful line from *Ash Wednesday*: 'Teach us to care and not to care.' If I can find it, being able to feel 'I couldn't care less' is the best antidote to my insomnia, and to simply say to the demon, 'Don't be silly.'

z z z z

Insomniacs only dream they're awake ...

Top ten mantras

Keep these thoughts in focus and they will help you keep your insomnia in perspective, and may make the world seem not so bad after all.

1. You get more sleep than you think.
2. It is a myth that we need 8 hours' sleep. Well-being can be had for much less.
3. Poor sleep does not make you more unhealthy or more prone to serious illness. As long as you can get some sleep and relax your body, you will be fine.
4. We don't need to recover all our lost sleep, or to recover as much sleep as we think we do.
5. A positive attitude is as good as a good night's sleep.
6. Rest assured: your body knows how to sleep. The ability to sleep well is innate, a gift we all possess and never lose.
7. Sleep problems are not solved with the intellect. It's your subconscious that knows you best, and who will right it for you.
8. Don't let the day be the build-up to the night; and don't let the night rule your day.
9. Be at peace with your insomnia, especially at night.
10. Think management, not cure. The cure will follow effortlessly.

Phase Three:
Getting further help –
orthodox and
complementary treatments
and techniques

Insomnia is complicated stuff, and it's no wonder that we are pre-pared to try anything that may help. I will readily admit to being a 'therapy junkie'. What I have discovered is that every practitioner has a slightly different spin on the causes of – and therefore the treatment for – insomnia; hopefully the following pages will help you kick-start the kind of therapy that is right for you.

Sleep scientists will hotly disagree, but don't make the mistake of necessarily seeking expert help with a complete cure in mind. If that comes, it'll be the icing on the cake and it could save you a lot of disappointment and frustration on the way. Like everything to do with insomnia, however, if you lower your sights, ironically you've probably got more chance of success. Even if a treatment doesn't cure your insomnia, it should definitely help, and where comple-mentary therapies are concerned may enrich you in other ways that you hadn't even bargained for.

When it comes to medical practitioners, orthodox or otherwise, we are not used to, nor are good at, asking questions: doctor knows best, and the patient's role is to take the advice/medicine gratefully. Where insomnia is concerned, though, it's often the other way round. Don't be afraid to ask questions. You could be saving both of your time and money.

z z z z

Orthodox vs complementary medicine

Orthodox treatments (medical doctors/sleep disorder centres and clinics/drugs) are symptom-led – that is, they will attempt to tackle your insomnia head-on, with the hope and expectation of curing your symptoms. If you see a sleep-disorder specialist, you will probably be recommended some kind of sleep-restriction regime (discussed on page 200) to help get your sleep back on track.

Complementary practitioners take a different route. They are primarily in the business of healing. Their approach is holistic – they look at the whole person – and they work to correct overall imbalances and re-establish homeostasis so the body can then heal itself. Indeed, 'rebalancing' is the single word you will most hear. The London Sleep Centre (page 190) tries to bridge the gap between the two and is one place which is adamant that there are effective cures for insomnia; for chronic insomniacs, who have already tried everything, belts-and-braces specialist help from a sleep clinic may be the answer.

Both approaches have a high degree of success. It's up to you which you explore. Nor are the two mutually exclusive – most of us will try a mixture at some time. As a good friend pointed out, curing is short term, healing is long term: some people say it never stops.

Seeking expert help – dos and don'ts

- Do your homework first, and take your time in deciding which of the various therapies to try.
- If you want to try conventional medical help, be prepared to be persistent or go private. In the UK, for example, all specialist help, NHS or private, will require referral from your GP – so he or she is the person you need to convince.
- Recommendation from someone who knows you well, or whom you trust, is usually the best route to finding a complementary practitioner who will be right for you. In addition, often one therapist may be able to recommend other suitable therapists.

- It is very important to have faith in your therapist, and for your therapist to believe that he or she can genuinely help you alleviate your insomnia. It is a proven and well-accepted fact that success or failure can depend on this as much as the treatment offered, be this from a conventional or complementary practitioner. (Such is the power of the placebo effect that drug companies dismiss 30 per cent of positive results in trials, because they know that if a patient *believes* a drug will work, this can have more of an effect than the drug itself.)
- Always ask how long it should take for you to see improvement. Often it will not be possible to tell you, but ask anyway.
- It's important to give a particular therapy a fair trial. If, after that, it is not producing the desired results or making you feel better in some way, it's time to move on.
- If you want to, say, combine hypnotherapy with homoeopathy or chiropractic care and sleeping pills or reflexology, check with the practitioner(s) first. It may be a good idea, but it may not.
- Make sure you tell the practitioner anything else you're trying, including medications, supplements, herbal remedies, relaxation techniques and dietary changes.
- Do a sleep diary (see page 287) for a week before you go for your first appointment. You will be able to articulate your sleep problem much better, and it may give the practitioner important clues as to how to treat it.

The medical health care service

The general medical profession receives minimal training on sleep disorders and insomnia, yet it is your family doctor you are likely to go to first. Moreover, in the UK, if you want orthodox treatment you have no option but to start with your GP; that's the way the system works. Indeed, concerns over lack of sleep are among the most common complaints that all family doctors hear. Most, frankly, are not able to assist that much. It is well known that being faced with an insomniac or anyone with severe sleeping problems is one of most clinicians' worst nightmares, as they feel powerless to do anything. As a result, over 80 per cent of people suffering from insomnia go undetected, or are not diagnosed effectively, and it is one of the few complaints that doctors will let the patient diagnose for themselves. Like Dorothy, below, chronic insomniacs are sometimes presumed to have some sort of psychological disorder, so get shunted off to a therapist without having the benefit of a specialist diagnosis provided by sleep-disorder centres and clinics.

Understandably, increasingly general practitioners are reluctant to prescribe sleeping pills, especially for anyone experiencing long-term problems with sleep. The usual treatment, therefore, is anti-depressants first; followed by sleeping pills as a fall-back strategy (see page 204). That said, every year over 20 million sleeping pills are prescribed. Make sure you really want and need them first.

Dorothy's story – The stoic insomniac

Dorothy, 58, works as a practice director in her husband's accountancy firm and has suffered from insomnia for over 20 years. Like many insomniacs, she has sought help from her doctor, but finds herself still floundering and putting up with the problem as best she can.

> With me, it's worry that keeps me awake. I fall asleep easily, sleep for three hours, then wake up around 1–2ish, alert. My brain is as bright as a button. I immediately start to worry about any problems about the previous day – even if there are none, I create them for myself. I never think about anything else in the night, just these worries. It's like I have a need to put the world to rights. I write them down – I can write reams at times, and will keep them to refer back to if they're important problems – for example, at work or with the family.
>
> I try breathing exercises for an hour or so – we have a soothing music tape which helps as well, but if I can't get back to sleep, which is usually the case, I get up and go to a spare room, do a bit of reading, open up my briefcase, or sometimes will do some ironing. I don't really like doing this, but it's a question of having to, and it's not fair to disturb my husband's sleep.

My concentration at work is not as good as I'd like. Often I'll get a better night's sleep on Friday evenings, and will nap for an hour after lunch at weekends.

I slept fine until I was made chairman of the school governors in the early 1980s – I was afraid of the responsibility, starting waking up, and it's been the same ever since.

The doctor has tried to give me sleeping pills but I've always resisted them. A couple of years ago I had a mini-breakdown, and was sent to my local psychotherapy consultant for one-to-one counselling and group therapy, though I can't say it helped much. My doctor wants me to go back again but I'm not sure. I'd really like to do something about my insomnia, but don't know how or where to go next. I've heard of sleep clinics but my doctor tells me he doesn't know of any.

Sleep clinics and advisory services

Sleep clinics and sleep-disorder centres are where you go for profes-sional medical treatment by doctors and consultants who specialize in sleep disorders, including insomnia, and where medical research (sleep laboratories) on sleep is carried out. It ought to be easy to find out about them, but generally it isn't. The US has a good network up and running (see Directory, page 240), but in the UK GPs don't generally seem to know they exist, and NHS sleep laboratories and clinics don't usually have the facilities to deal with the public direct. Happily, however, things are changing. The British Sleep Society (page 268) recently conducted a comprehensive survey on 'UK Sleep Service Providers' (currently there are over 150) which has been sent to all GP Primary Care Trusts. The survey details which disorders the sleep centre specializes in, including insomnia, whether they are happy to receive referrals from a GP, the treatment facilities they offer, whether they treat adults and/or children, and whether any of the consultants or staff accept private patients. Very few specialize in insomnia, but at least it's a start for your doctor. If he or she isn't aware of this survey, the British Sleep Society will forward a copy: tell your doctor to e-mail: bssoffice@huntingdon52freeserve.co.uk. Otherwise, you can call NHS Direct on 0845 4647, who are very helpful, will take your details, do their best to find sleep centres near you, and either call back or write to you. They will also send you useful advice and a useful little booklet, *How to Cope with Sleep*, published by Mind (National Association for Mental Health). On-line, you can either key in something like 'UK sleep clinics' or 'UK private sleep clinics' on a search engine – you'll get back over 1,000 references – or you can go to: www.neuronic.com/bss/sleep%20contacts.htm, which has its own incomplete but useful list. Note, too, that in the UK sleep research laboratories do not usually treat patients, though individual consultants may hold private clinics. Like any sleep clinic anywhere in the world, however, they often need sleep-deprived volunteers – worth checking out if you have one in your area.

Private sleep clinics are similarly difficult to track down. In the UK, The London Sleep Centre in Harley St (www.londonsleepcentre.co.uk) is the newest, brightest and a real step forward in terms of a joined-up approach to the treatment of insomnia and other sleep disorders, utilizing rigorous scientific assessments and treatments coupled with behavioural and complementary therapies such as acupuncture. Take a look at their excellent website and you can't help but be encouraged that there is a solution (and will want to book in straightaway).

Whichever country you live in, it's often possible to pay for treatment under private healthcare insurance schemes – ask the clinic concerned. For UK readers, Some BUPA hospitals also treat sleep disorders (see page 270).

Outside the UK, if your family doctor doesn't know of any, your best bet is to search the web for a medical sleep association you can contact for help.

Sleep clinics: What they do

Most of us only hear about sleep clinics in the press or through movies (www.amazon.com has a selection), or novels such as *The House of Sleep* by Jonathan Coe. What can you expect? What you don't do (which is what I expected when I went), is automatically get swept off to the sleep lab and wired up. As Simone de Lacey,

z z z z

Principal Technologist and manager of Guy's and St Thomas' Sleep Disorders Centre in London, explains, each centre's approach and treatments vary, but will always begin with a detailed consultation. There may then be various tests, including blood and hormone tests, or the use of state-of-the-art electronic monitoring such as an actigraph (a wristwatch-like device that measures your daily life activity and helps determine any unusual circadian rhythms or day-time napping). You may be asked to complete a sleep diary. Given that insomnia inevitably impinges on your mental and emotional well-being, you can expect to fill in questionnaires relating to your mental state and quality of life. Rarely, you may be asked to spend a night in a sleep laboratory – more comfy than it sounds – to undergo a complete polysomnographic study in order to assess the quality and quantity of your sleep, and whether there are any physical reasons why your sleep may be disturbed, such as teeth-grinding, sleep apnoea, restless legs, etc. In the last 15 years, refer-rals at Guy's and St Thomas' Sleep Disorder Centre have shot up from 50 to 1,500 per year, which gives you a measure of just how chronic lack of sleep is becoming.

Sleep Matters: Insomnia Helpline (UK)

Part of the Medical Advisory Service, which gives help on a variety of health problems, including insomnia, this helpline is manned by friendly nurses who will listen to your sleep problem, be it insom-nia, snoring or restless legs, and refer you to the appropriate organization. You may find you know as much as they do, that you've been there, done that, but it's still nice to talk. They also pro-duce their own Sleep Matters newsletter. Send SAE to PO Box 3087, London W4 4ZP. Tel: 0208 994 9874. Lines are open Monday to Friday and Sunday from 6–10 p.m.

For internet chat forums and remedyline.com, see page 238.

Sleep Assessment and Advisory Service

This is the equivalent of an insomniac's knight in shining armour, providing what many of us who have tried everything want and need most: a fast track to an independent qualified sleep expert who understands insomnia. Run personally by Professor Chris

zzzz

Idzikowski, specifically for those suffering from insomnia and non-respiratory sleep problems and disorders, the service (available worldwide) provides a unique private telephone consultation service. You book an appointment, discuss your case with Professor Idzikowski direct, and receive a follow-up letter outlining suggested treatment, etc. For those who require it, a further on-line sleep-management service is available, using sleep diaries; the Service will also provide letters for doctors if further medical treatment is required. They will usually ask you to complete their sleep diary before consultation. This can be found on www.sleepspecialist.co.uk/d5.htm.

The current cost is £50 per consultation, plus a modest weekly or monthly charge for additional on-line support, which is far cheaper than going private, and may be all you need.

I cannot recommend this service highly enough. It changed my views on sleep-restriction therapy (page 200) and gives every insomniac or anyone who is sleeping badly the opportunity to try it under expert guidance, simply and easily. Telephone 0845 1300 933, or e-mail: office@sleepspecialist.co.uk.

My case

By the time I'd found the Sleep Advisory Service, I figured I understood my insomnia pretty well, and had been through everything on the Master Plan and most therapies. After completing their sleep diary for 10 days, I was provisionally diagnosed as suffering from:

- Psychophysiological (conditioned) insomnia
- Phase-advance syndrome (or at least a tendency for early morning awakening)
- Sleeping pill dependence

At this moment your state is even more muddled because of what you are trying to do with writing a book. You need to be an observer to see how various 'treatments' work, but at the same time you are emotionally entangled with your condition. Sleep is certainly one of those states that as you focus on it you become unlikely to evoke it (hence all the therapies that belong to the 'zap it' category, e.g. alcohol, sleeping pills; or the 'look away'/distract/displacement' therapies).

There is a possibility of mild hypomania-depression, which could provoke periods of insomnia coupled with early morning awakening. Or, on the same track, your brain is just a little hyper-arousable. However, first things first – it's time for a regime.

I was then advised the following:

- 'Regularity is extremely important for sleep and how it ties in with the light-dark cycle. Given you have larkish tendencies, you should go to bed at: 22:00.'
- 'Some sleep restriction to increase "sleep pressure". Get up at 05:00.'
- 'The 20-minute rule – if in bed for longer than 20 minutes awake, quietly go to another "rest/sleep" location. Do nothing there other than waiting to feel when you feel sleepy. Don't DO anything other than observing how you feel. Be comfortable. Lights off, no radio, darkness. If you feel sleepy, return to your bed. Keep repeating this during the night BUT if you have been up and down three times, then abandon the attempt to sleep in your own bed, just rest/sleep in your alternative resting place.'
- 'Ideally, no medications, no other methods to try to actively do something about your sleep.'

Going to bed at 10 p.m. was no problem, but even though my final waking was 4.45-5 a.m. on the dot, as daylight broke (it was May), it was too much of a struggle to get up then. We changed to 10.30 p.m. bed, and 5.30 a.m. get up. The regime suited me: my sleep gradually became less disruptive and I had gained 2–3 hours' extra day time, albeit at a gentle half-awake potter. I continued to live the life of a monk, faded early evening, kept my usual ritual of hot baths, candles, soothing music and viniyoga exercises before going to bed, and fell asleep most nights easily for the first time in a long time. I never did manage the 20-minute rule.

Bright light therapy

We've all heard of light boxes to boost serotonin levels to overcome SAD (Seasonal Affective Disorder), which makes people despondent or depressed during the winter months because of the lack of sunlight. Using bright light to overcome circadian rhythm sleep disorders, and reset your circadian pacemaker back to normal, is also common practice, and works – not just for people with sleep disorders but for shift-workers, too.

It's based on the principle that bright light in the evening tends to slow the body clock down, while bright light in the morning tends to speed it up. For the two specific disorders below, where either the time you go to sleep or the time you wake up is typically three hours later or earlier than normal, it can provide a more effective therapy than drugs, simply because it's treating the cause, rather than the symptoms. For it to work, you have to use properly timed bright light for a specified amount of time every day. The science and application of bright light therapy is relatively new, hence is not yet fixed, but broadly it works like this:

Can't get to sleep, won't go to sleep

Insomniacs who can't get to sleep, and find it difficult to stay asleep, or night owls who can't go to bed until the early hours of the morning and can't get up until much later than most of us (common amongst teenagers), are usually suffering from Delayed Sleep Phase Syndrome (DSPS). This means their body clock is permanently lagging behind normal. Here, sitting in front of bright light in the morning, on waking, for up to 2 hours, advances the body clock, fast-forwarding it to normal, thus allowing you to sleep and get up at 'normal' times.

Waking up too early

For insomniacs who, like me, are wide awake before the larks (common also amongst the elderly), or for people who can go to sleep but can't stay asleep, and wake up very early, the opposite applies. Often the problem here is Advance Sleep Phase Syndrome (ASPS), which means their body clocks are running faster than normal. Bright light

z z z z

in the evening slows the body clock down, pulling it [...] mal, thus allowing people to sleep longer. Studies show tha[...] as 30 minutes in the evening, for example, can minimize early morning insomnia, though some patients need much longer.

Light boxes mimic the intensity of natural sunlight, are not especially expensive, and are easy to use. They vary in intensity from 2,500–10,000 lux, the equivalent of a cloudy-bright day. The stronger the intensity, the less time you need to use the box for. For anyone who finds the dark days of winter difficult, suffers from jet-lag or does shift-work (see David's story on page 45), they are a good idea. I'm using a travel-lite model, and don't find the light obtrusive at all.

For insomnia, the science is both new and quite complicated, so consult expert advice first and check that it is medically OK for you to use one. For example, the three sleep drivers – body temperature, serotonin and melatonin – are all regulated by light. How much dark you get is as critical as how much light (ASPSs should avoid early-morning light). Nor is it a quick fix – allow up to three months for significant improvement.

Light boxes are used in exactly the same way to treat jet-lag, and can also be effective for more generalized insomnia. The SAD Light Box company (www.sad.uk.com), one of the major UK specialists, are happy to give advice. For details, see the Directory, page 252.

Nor does light therapy stop with light boxes. The American company Bio-Brite Inc. offer a wide range of all kinds of light therapy and jet-lag products, including light visors, light windows, desk lamps and sunrise clocks. For more, see www.biobrite.com. For more on how light regulates sleep, see page 18.

Using bright light therapy to manage jet-lag

Jet-lag is a self-induced jumbling up of circadian rhythms. You may be able to cross time zones in minutes, but your body clock can't. The very thought of it is enough to make an insomniac postpone a holiday. Generally you need about a day for each time zone crossed to re-establish your body clock; you can cope with up to 3 hours' time difference, but as we know it gets increasingly difficult after that. Alternatively, you can use bright light to help reset your body clock.

Perversely, it's light either at night or very early in the morning that counts, not in the middle of the day. The principle is exactly the same as above: Bright light in the evening will delay your wake-up time; bright light very early in the morning will bring the body clock forward so you wake up earlier. To achieve maximum effect in the shortest possible time, exposure to bright light must correspond either side of your lowest body temperature – about 4 a.m. for normal sleepers. Bright light immediately before 4 a.m. will delay the clock, helpful for going West; bright light between 4 and 6 a.m. will bring it forwards, helpful when travelling East. The problem of course is the 4 a.m bit: science and living a real life are not always happy bedfellows.

As far as your body clock is concerned, flying West to East, when you are going backwards in time (hence artificially extending the day) is always easier than flying East to West, when you are artificially shortening the day. The reason is simple. It's easier for most people to go to sleep if their body clock says it's really late, than to stay up if it says it's really early. The penny is beginning to drop. In the US, for example, The Hilton Hotel Corporation have equipped some of their hotels with special 'sleep-tight' rooms containing light boxes, earplugs, etc.

Jet-lag (and shift-work) are relatively modern phenomena which need to be taken seriously, particularly by employers, who often don't do nearly enough for their sleep-deprived employees. If you need to cross three or more time zones, the clearest and most sensible advice on using sunlight comes from the book *Beating Insomnia*, and goes like this:

1. Normal sleepers (i.e., those whose waking time is normally around 7 a.m.):
   Travelling east: avoid light between 3.30 and 8.30 a.m., then look for bright light until 11.30 p.m.
   Travelling west: bright light between 21.30 p.m. and 00.30 a.m; avoid bright light until 4.30 p.m. and thereafter.

z z z z

2. Owls and larks (i.e. normal waking time earlier or later than 7 a.m.):
Adjust the above times accordingly – if your habitual waking time is 9 a.m. (owl), you would avoid bright light after travelling east from 5.30–10.30 a.m.; if your normal waking time is 5 a.m. (lark), you would avoid bright light between 01.30 and 6.30 a.m. Similarly, if travelling west you would move the recommended periods of getting and avoiding bright light forwards or back by two hours.

Jet-lag and products to help manage it, including watches, are becoming big business. For the latest info, see www.jetlagsolutions.com and www.biobrite.com. For details of the UK Jetlag clinic, see page 269.

Rio Lightmask™

One of the latest light-therapy devices, developed in the late 1980s by research neurologist Dr Duncan Andersen as a treatment for migraines, the Rio Lightmask™ has also been found to alleviate insomnia and PMS in some people. Trials in Australia on war veterans unable to sleep, for example, reported significant improvement. Other users report deeper sleep and feeling less muddled and clearer on waking. It's also good for jet-lag.

It works by shining a pulsed light into your eyes whilst your eyes are closed. Why it works is still not fully understood, but is likely to do with the connection between the optic nerve and its influence on the suprachiasmatic nucleus and pineal gland (see page 20).

You use the mask in bed, to help you get to sleep or get back to sleep. The mask is comfortable and easy to use. However, the shock of having bright light beamed into your eyes (even while they are closed) is unnerving and disorientating, at least initially. You can fine-tune the programme to suit you, but if, like me, you just can't stand light of any kind when it's dark, the mask is unlikely to be suitable for you. For everyone else, it's worth a try (the curative power of light is one of the latest and potentially most exciting fields of healthcare). It comes with a money-back guarantee. For more, see www.lightmask.com. Also available from Rio Beauty (see Directory, page 248): www.riobeauty.com.

Cognitive behavioural therapy

This technique, developed over 20 years ago, has been one of the most successful in treating chronic insomnia. It is widely used in the US, where it has been shown to help at least a third of insomniacs become normal sleepers, with 70–80 per cent reporting that they've derived benefit from the treatment. It is also used in sleep clinics in the UK.

CBT is based on the belief that much of insomnia is learned negative thoughts and behaviour. Like all good therapies, it takes an integrated approach, focusing on four key areas:

a) Tackling and modifying stressful negative and often inaccurate thoughts about sleep. For examples, see pages 179 and 184.
b) Addressing bad sleeping habits, such as spending too much time in bed relative to actual sleep time. See below.
c) Incorporating relaxation techniques to improve relaxation skills. See page 146.
d) Identifying and improving lifestyle habits. See pages 38, 101 and 107.

Cognitive behavioural therapy forms the basis of Dr Greg Jacob's book *Say Goodnight to Insomnia*; the website www.talkaboutsleep.com contains his six-week self-help CBT programme which you can download.

Reorganizing sleep time

It's very easy when you don't sleep to end up with haphazard, erratic sleep regimes, and to be undisciplined about the time you go to bed and the time you spend in bed. Some of us love our beds and can't wait to get to bed despite how little sleep we may have had the night before; others may have grown to hate our beds and put off bed-time for as long as we can. Still others lie in when we can, on the off-chance we may catch another scrap of sleep. This is especially so at the weekends, and leads to the phenomenon which affects normal sleepers as well as poor sleepers: Sunday Night Insomnia.

z z z z

Ironically, we are making it worse for ourselves. Establishing a regular sleep regime is sacrosanct in sleep therapy, and altering the time you go to bed and being disciplined about the time you stay in bed are two keystone techniques used by sleep specialists to get your sleep back on track. This includes weekends as well as weekdays. Your body clock gets resynchronized with the sleep-awake cycle every night, and even minor changes can affect it negatively. Don't panic, though – these are temporary techniques, quite specific in their intent. As soon as your sleep patterns improve, and you can manage your sleep better, you can afford to take a more relaxed approach, though – because they make such good sleep-management sense – you will probably want to build them into your life.

Step one: a regular routine

This means not just going to bed at approximately the same time every night, but getting up at the same time as well, irrespective of how poor your sleep has been. It's the getting-up-at-the-same-time which is the key. The circadian rhythm needs one fixed point to stabilize itself around. The theory being you can't control or predict the time you fall asleep, but you can control the time you get up. It applies to weekends, too, because every time you sleep in, you delay the rise in your body temperature, which means you delay the time you are likely to get to sleep the following night, thus running the risk of upsetting all the good work you have put in the previous week at better regulating your sleep. Think of sleeping in as 'mini jet-lag', which is effectively what it is.

It sounds very simple, but comes more easily to some than others, especially if you share your life with someone who has an entirely different sleep routine. The getting-up-earlier bit is easy in summer, but can be more difficult in winter, though if you are the kind of insomniac who can't face getting up in the middle of the night to 'do something useful', it works well. A new day always seems more hopeful than fumbling around in the middle of yesterday's night, and if you do train yourself to get up within half an hour of your final waking, you do feel really pleased with yourself.

Plus it is amazing how much you can accomplish in those quiet early hours.

This step has two other advantages. Getting up at a different time to your loved one is generally more acceptable than going to bed at a seriously different time; and you don't feel half as guilty or frustrated when you start to get tired in the early evening. All of a sudden it's natural to do so, because you've already had a long and more productive day, so you can feel good about being tired instead of feeling downcast and frustrated. I also found, initially at least, that it miraculously took the pressure off sleeping. Because it automatically compresses the time you naturally have to sleep, it sort of sends out a cue to your brain to get on with it. Whereas if you know you have oceans of time – the normal safety net for not sleeping – your brain doesn't need to get on with it, so doesn't.

For insomniac owls it's going to bed later than they did previously that can often work. I know one insomniac owl who worked at a sleep lab and thought not going to bed until 3 a.m. was the best thing he'd ever discovered. A couple more tips from *Say Goodnight to Insomnia:*

- Go to bed and get up at the same time. Stay within the 30 minutes of the same rising time every day, even if it means putting the alarm clock on.
- If you must (occasionally) sleep in, limit it to one hour; get some bright light as soon as you get up, and compensate by going to bed one hour later that night.

Step two: sleep-restriction therapy

Sleep scientists have one rule of thumb: the earlier you get up and the later you go to bed, the higher the probability you will sleep, and the better quality your sleep will be – that is, you will fall asleep more quickly, have less interrupted sleep, more deep sleep, and sleep longer. This is because the longer you are awake, the greater the pressure from your brain to get to sleep!

Sleep experts use *sleep efficiency* to determine how successful, sleepwise, your time in bed is. To measure this you simply divide

z z z z

time spent asleep by time spent in bed, and multiply by a hundred. People who literally use bed for sleep, or rather spend most of their time in bed asleep, have a high sleep efficiency, around 90 per cent. Insomniacs typically spend at least a third of the time in bed thrashing around being awake, and therefore we have much lower sleep efficiencies, around 65 per cent or less. And because we spend so much of our time in bed awake, bed for us often gets distorted as a cue for being awake rather than, as for everyone else, being asleep.

To alter this, and change your perception so that bed equals sleep rather than non-sleep, you need to raise your sleep efficiency, which is what sleep-restriction therapy is all about. If the discipline of rescheduling your sleep time to a regular bedtime, and getting up earlier, haven't helped, then this is the next step. If your insomnia or sleeplessness is not that severe, it should be fairly straightforward, albeit drastic for a few weeks. If you are working, and worry about the effect it may have on your work (even though it probably won't have one), you may want to wait until you've got some time off before you give it a try.

The aim is to reduce the time you spend in bed so that it more closely matches the time you are asleep. This is the official version of what you do:

- Use a sleep diary to track your sleep for one week, and calculate how many hours of sleep you average per night (there's no point guessing or relying on memory).
- Add one hour and make that the *maximum* time you spend in bed. Unless you are practising under the supervision of a sleep expert, some sleep scientists advise making the total time in bed no fewer than $5^1/2$ hours, to ensure you have the opportunity of getting a full quota of core sleep (wish!!).
- Start with your getting-up time, using your natural pattern, and work backwards. Thus, if your maximum allowed time in bed works out at $5^1/2$ hours, and you want or need to get up at 6.30 a.m., you don't get in bed before 1 a.m., no matter how tired you feel.
- Once your sleep efficiency has improved to around 85 per cent for two weeks, you then increase your time in bed by 15

minutes per week, by going to bed 15 minutes earlier – but be sure to get up at the same time. If your sleep efficiency falls, then you go back and repeat the process until it's re-established again.

It usually takes around 2–4 weeks to show improvement, so don't expect overnight miracles, and though initially you may be getting (or will feel you're getting) less sleep, you will get more sleep in the long run. It's common to feel drowsy when you first start: this is a sign it is working. Also, you are getting more deep sleep, which eventually will lead you to feeling more refreshed.

The alternative approach: 'halfway house' restriction therapy

Sharp – or should I say bleary-eyed? – insomniacs like me, for whom even 1–2 hours' unbroken sleep is a luxury, 5 hours' total sleep a rarity, and 3–4 hours' sleep nearer the norm, will quickly calculate that the amount of rescheduling they are required to do is as frighteningly drastic as going cold turkey is for a smoker or alcoholic. Asking larks to go to bed at 3 a.m., or owls to get up at 5 a.m., is like putting us on the rack and turning the screws. Unless you are under the guidance of a sleep expert, who can motivate you and work out precisely what is best for you, a more pragmatic approach to sleep-restriction therapy is to modify it according to your body-clock and personality. As Professor Chris Idzikowski comfortingly said to me, 'Gently does it is always a good rule.' True. I'm a lark, and getting up earlier than I wanted worked brilliantly, but as someone who can't pass a bed after 9 p.m. and not want to jump in, hanging around until I was dog-tired and going to bed much later, didn't.

If you're trying sleep restriction on your own and can't face cold turkey, take a slightly more benign approach, teasing your insomnia apart into what you know you can cope with:

- Decide whether you're a lark or owl, and check out how you feel about what changing your bedtime says to you.
- Calculate the average number of hours you normally sleep, as before.

$z^z{}_z{}^z$

- Change your wake-up time as much as you can realistically manage, working backwards as before, but allowing for your body-clock and your feelings. Larks will respond to getting up earlier; owls can compensate by staying up later.
- You may need to juggle with the going-to-bed/getting-up times to find the best compromise that you can manage comfortably.

This has worked really well for me, enabling me to fall asleep without difficulty most nights, and in the main to get a good chunk of sleep when it matters most, early on in the night. It is also the case that if I stray from the regime, and go back to my old erratic patterns, falling asleep starts getting difficult again. As falling asleep is the critical confidence-boosting button for me, this means having to start the process all over again. The moral being: stick at it, or get an expert to guide you through.

Step three: getting out of bed

Another Holy Cow. Every sleep expert is adamant that you do *not* lie awake in the middle of the night tossing and turning in bed; you get up, go to another room and do something menial or relaxing, or just sit there, until your eyelids start to droop. Only then do you return to your bed. And you keep doing this every time you wake up and can't get back to sleep within a few minutes. The rationale is to associate bed with sleep, not with being awake. As noted above, being awake is something you are somewhere else, not in your bed. Professor Jim Horne at Loughborough Sleep Centre recommends doing a jigsaw puzzle – a good idea, and far more appealing than ironing. Light reading or listening to music or tapes are the other activities usually recommended.

This is fine, and works for many people, but not all. For example, I like my bed, and hate getting out of it in the night. Panic sets in that I'm going to wake myself up even more, especially if I have to put on a light. I also feel more vulnerable out of bed than in, so I prefer to stay put and be peaceful and do some relaxation exercises or listen to tapes.

Other insomniacs I've discussed this with are split equally down the middle. Some think it's great; others, like me, think it's daft. It all depends on how you view your bed and how relaxed or restless you are in the dark hours (getting up if you're wide awake obviously makes more sense than if you feel you're a nod away from dozing off). Like every piece of good advice about insomnia or sleeplessness, it's only good if it suits you – though don't expect medical sleep experts necessarily to agree.

Bootzin stimulus control

Developed 20 years ago by American sleep scientist Richard Bootzin to counteract conditioned insomnia, this method is somewhat draconian, but simple:

1. Only go to bed when you're sleepy.
2. Only use bed for sleep (or sex).
3. If you can't sleep after 10–20 minutes, get up and go to another room.
4. Only go back to bed when you're sleepy.
5. Keep repeating step 3 as necessary, every time you wake in the night.

If your problem is not being able to fall asleep, you add:
6. Set the alarm for the same time every day, and get up when it goes off.
7. Don't nap.

Sleeping pills

Sleeping pills offer a temporary crutch. Ironically, though millions are prescribed every year, for insomniacs they are often a last resort. No one wants to take them, for all sorts of understandable reasons, not least the fear that once you start, you'll never be able to stop. Sleep scientists are divided. Some advocate them, others do not. Doctors are also very reticent to prescribe sleeping pills for insomniacs. Initially you are much more likely to be offered an anti-depressant, which is perceived as a lower-risk and makes the doctor (and the patient, sometimes) apprehensive.

There are many heartbreaking stories of insomniacs who have been taking sleeping pills for several years. However, it's too easy to say people get addicted to sleeping pills. Nicotine and caffeine are as physically addictive, or even more so, than many modern sleeping pills. Speaking as one who lived on them for six months, what you get addicted to is being able to sleep, to have that break from yourself and having the responsibility for getting yourself to sleep taken from you. That's why sleeping pills are bliss. And why they become a trap. It's a psychological addiction as much as a physical one. If you do consider them, make sure you learn a little bit about them first.

There was a time when I refused to use them, a time when I couldn't face going to bed without them, and a time when I swore I would never take another one again. Until I signed up with the Sleep Assessment Advisory Service (page 191) I had come full circle, and was using them very occasionally as an emergency and effective aid which gave me sleep when I was desperate and knew that I needed some help to keep me on track physically, mentally and emotionally. Like other post-sleeping pill dependents I've talked to, I often went weeks or months without taking any. Nor do I feel guilty or inadequate any more because I might use them.

Changing my approach and being absolutely strict with their use (the difficult and disciplined but crucial bit) at the time seemed to me – and still seems – a sensible compromise. That said, as more than one sleep doctor has explained, sleeping pill and post-sleeping pill dependents are the most difficult group to treat, particularly high-dose benzodiazepine users. If you are or have been dependent on sleeping pills for some time, you will almost certainly need expert help and support to wean yourself off them. Even mild one-time users are better advised to keep off them if possible. As a post-sleeping pill dependent, The Sleep Assessment and Advisory Service advised I switched to something like Nytol (see page 208) if I was desperate. Thus far I have managed to stick with this approach.

What prescription sleeping pills do

Sleeping pills do not cure insomnia. They are a highly targeted, highly specific quick fix, the equivalent of bringing in the Special Squad. They don't help you become a normal sleeper, and they only tackle the symptoms, not the underlying cause, of your sleeplessness. They work on the brain, not the body, depressing its activity by slowing down brainwaves. They relieve anxiety, relax muscles and induce sleep. The difference between the various brands is usually the time it takes for the effects to wear off – that is, the time it takes the body to break them down and get them out of your system, known as the 'half-life'. This can be anything from a few hours to days. Brands with a short half-life stay in the body for less time than brands with a long half-life; the longer they hang around, the more likely you are to experience drowsiness or other side-effects – which is why you need to know exactly what they do, and for how long.

As cited in *Beating Insomnia*, the two classes of sleeping pills most commonly prescribed today are benzodiazepines (BZs) such as temazepam (Restoril), flurazepam (Dalmane) and lorazepam (Ativan), and the 'non-benzodiazepine benzodiazepines' (imidazopyridines and cyclopyrrolones) such as zolpidem (Ambein, Stilnoct), zalepon (Sonata) and zoplicone (Imovane).

Barbituates, responsible for several high-profile suicides in the 1960s and 1970s – including that of Marilyn Monroe and Jimi Hendrix – are nasty, old-fashioned, stronger and more addictive: Don't take them.

Benzodiazepines

These are also muscle-relaxants. Dependence can result with long-term, high-dose use. Short-term use can cause rebound wakefulness.

Imidazopyridines and Cyclopyrrolones

These newer compounds affect the same sites in the brain as BZs, but belong to a different chemical class. They are shorter acting, with lower risk of daytime sedation or rebound wakefulness.

What are their effects?

A sleeping pill will not necessarily give you eight hours' sleep. In fact, they will almost certainly give you less; anti-sleeping pill sleep scientists also point out they often don't give you more than you could expect anyway. This is because most new-generation sleeping pills are best at knocking you out and putting you to sleep. They are not particularly effective at relieving repeated waking, or early waking, and generally don't last more than four hours. Occasional use of these sleeping pills is unlikely to have any side-effects, except a quick burst of morning-after euphoria the next day. Continued use is different. Memory, concentration and general mental alertness can all suffer. It's like being 'fogged up'. You don't seem to be able to make connections as fast, and become duller and dumber in the process. For me, it was like having early senile dementia. Other common side-effects run the gamut from headaches and nausea to nightmares.

Sleeping pills increase Stage 2, or light sleep, but lessen deep sleep and REM sleep (which is why often you recall dreams much less on sleeping pills). This means that technically the quality of your sleep suffers, though you will not see it that way.

The longer you use sleeping pills, the more the brain becomes 'habituated' and the less effective they become. Their effectiveness usually lasts no more than 4–6 weeks with nightly use, sometimes less, and is why they are prescribed for no more than 1–3 weeks at a time. The answer is not to increase the dose, but to stop taking them, even though it will not be pleasant. The longer you take them, the more you also run the risk of rebound insomnia when you stop, and the more physically addictive they can become, perpetuating the spiral that you are desperate to get out of.

Different sleeping pills have slightly different effects; some do suit better than others. So, if you try one kind and don't get along with it, try another. I went through four before I found the one that suited me (Stilnoct). Children, pregnant women, or anyone trying to have a baby or breastfeeding should *never* be given sleeping pills; elderly people – who take them more than any other group – don't metabolize them as efficiently or quickly, and are thus more sensitive to side-effects. If you are addictive by nature, give them a wide berth if you can. Finally, don't take them with alcohol, which can exacerbate their side-effects, and don't take them if you are taking other medication without checking with your doctor first.

For first-hand accounts of using various sleeping pills, see www.remedyfind.com.

Anti-depressants

There are two sorts of anti-depressants: those like Prozac (SSRIs) are very specific in their action. They boost serotonin but have nothing to do with helping you sleep; indeed, they may cause disrupted sleep. The other type of anti-depressant, such as amitriptylines, though they also increase serotonin, are sedating anti-depressants which, if taken in very small doses, induce sleep. These work in exactly the same way as sleeping pills; many of them are indeed sleeping pills, and are prescribed as such, it's just that pharmaceutical companies choose to register them as anti-depressants rather than sleeping pills.

Sedating anti-depressants do not disrupt deep sleep, are not physically addictive and do not cause rebound insomnia, though they will give you a dry mouth, constipation and can cause the same general 'fog'. I didn't like them one bit, but they work for other people. Again, only you – in consultation with your doctor – can find out what's best for you.

Over-the-counter sleeping pills

These include brands like Nytol, Sleep-Eez and Sominex. The active ingredient in all of these are anti-histamines, usually found in cold and allergy remedies, which have sedative effects. Diphenhydramine is the most common of these. They don't put you to sleep, but do make you sufficiently drowsy to enable you to fall asleep faster. Like prescription sleeping pills, their effects wear off with continual use; they should only be used for a short time. They don't work for everyone, either. Unlike sleeping pills, their action is not specific – the drowsiness is a side-effect of their main action, which is why

z z z z

many sleeping experts think we are wasting our money on them. For many of us, myself included, who've tried all the herbal remedies they can think of, these are the next best soft option. If your insomnia is temporary they will probably do the job; if it's chronic, they will almost certainly not. For a while, Nytol gave me some much-needed relief, though personally I need to be acutely sleep-deprived before they work well for me. Because they take a long time to clear from the body, only take them just before you go to bed, not when you wake up during the night.

Though I've never experienced any side-effects, those reported include dry mouth, dizziness and blurred vision. Nor should they be taken, for example, by people with angina, glaucoma, urinary or prostate problems, or with medications to prevent nausea or travel sickness; so do check with your pharmacist or doctor first.

Sleeping pill know-how

If you are considering prescription sleeping pills, this is what you should do when seeing your doctor. If you do take them, always read the infuriatingly small print which comes with every pack, including the long list of all possible side-effects.

1. Describe your sleep problem precisely: Do you find it difficult to go to sleep? Do you wake up frequently? Do you wake up too early? If you are anxious or depressed, discuss this also.
2. Discuss whether sleeping pills or an anti-depressant would be more suitable. If you have decided you'd rather try sleeping pills, don't be palmed off with anti-depressants.
3. Check out the sleeping pill the doctor chooses, and ask him or her to read out the description in MIMS. Check out what type it is, whether it is designed to put you to sleep, stop you from waking up, etc, possible side-effects, and how long it is likely to be effective – that is, how many hours sleep can you expect?

z z z z

4. Check to see what dosages are available. Insist on the lowest-dose pack. This is because a) you don't want to get hooked on a higher dose (you can always increase the dose later on), and b) at some time or other you will need to wean yourself off them.

Using sleeping pills

- Always start with the lowest dose.
- Wean yourself off sleeping pills gradually by reducing the dose. Sometimes this will require cutting them in half, then a quarter, etc., as necessary. Note that most are as hard as nails, so that trying to bite them into bits is not as easy as it sounds. Prepare to have your bedroom littered with bits of white stuff.

Matthew's story – the straightforward insomniac

Matthew, 28, a media consultant, suffered from insomnia for several years, and is one example where drugs have helped. But, as in his case, the important thing is finding the right one for you.

I've never been a great sleeper, but it got really bad during finals at university. I then worried so much about not being able to sleep it became a self-fulfilling prophesy. Afterwards, I went away on holiday to Mexico for three months, thinking I'd sleep like a log – and it was worse than ever.

With me, it's not being able to get to sleep that's the problem. I'm an owl; my brain really comes alive at 10 p.m. and I can stay up all night, no problem. Once I get to sleep, I'm fine. I'd go to bed about 12.30 and just lie there until 3, 4 or 5 a.m. before I'd drop off, so most of the time I was managing on four hours or less sleep a night. This went on for years. I became a zombie, always too tired to do anything, never being able to plan, and always having to cancel going out or doing anything, even if I really wanted to do it. I lived in fear of what I would or wouldn't be able to do.

I'd been prescribed temazepam when I was at university, but it was awful for me. I zonked out for eight hours and woke feeling totally disorientated and not rested in any way.

z z z z

Eventually, in desperation I went back to the doctor, who gave me zoplicone [one of the non-benzodiazepine benzodiazepines, with the brand name Imovane]. They sorted me, and changed my life. I took them for about three months, gradually reducing the dose to half and then a quarter of a tablet. In the end they were probably placebo, but they gave me the confidence I needed, and acted as a safety net for me.

Now, I have the occasional bad nights but most of the time my sleep is fine. I'll drop off and sleep for six to seven hours, which is what I need. I don't worry about not being able to get to sleep any more, and being tired no longer rules my life. If I have a bad night, I won't take a pill at 3 a.m., but will have one the following night if I need it and can't get to sleep within half an hour.

Complementary therapies

There are over 100 different recognized complementary therapies. Given the nature of insomnia, that means one or probably several are likely to be beneficial. I have heard successful and unsuccessful reports about most of them, and though it may sound defeatist, what works for one person does not necessarily work for the next. This is because complementary therapy treats the dynamic that is You. Much more so than orthodox medicine, therefore, complementary therapy is one area where you need to be prepared for trial and error. Believe me, I've tried more than most. And as every therapist knows, it is also much more likely to open up the Pandora's box that is You than to stick a plaster on it.

At their core, too, all are a form of energy medicine, be it connecting with and re-establishing the body's own life-force, or drawing on the universal force or energies, or both. Though many are gaining credibility and respectability fast, what complementary therapies often lack is empirical double-blinded trials. They make up for this with testimonials. Take a look at www.remedyfind.com and you'll find that, interestingly, many score higher ratings than sleeping pills.

Complementary methods suit some people more than others: If you feel you've come home, and feel good in some way about having complementary therapy (I do), you tend to get hooked pretty quickly.

Just before you do, be aware that complementary medicine can be a bit like peeling an onion. Deal with one symptom (or one layer) and often another pops up that was being masked by the original symptom. Fixing one area can highlight weaknesses elsewhere. To use a silly example, the true cause of the pain in your elbow may be some toxin lodged in your nervous system, or the after-effects of a vaccine given in childhood. Complementary practitioners understand this well, and will use their judgement as to what priorities need to be addressed before they can get to your insomnia.

It's also easy to expect too much, and invest too much hope in complementary therapies. Cures do happen from time to time, but the everyday reality is somewhat different. As award-winning health journalist Susan Clark points out in *What Really Works*, the big problem is that there are no real enforceable regulations, policing or monitoring of practitioners – anyone can take a course and set up shop. For this reason, take the tips on page 186 seriously.

A brief taster of what you can expect follows, together with a general what-can-help list. The A–Z of complementary therapies section in *What Really Works* gives you the ups and downs of most of them, and saves reading a book on each one. Susan Clark's website www.whatreallyworks.co.uk (e-mail: susan@whatreallyworks.co.uk) has an active chat line, info on most therapies and remedies, and useful advice on insomnia, too.

For more on vibrational (energy) medicine and the complementary therapies which are based on it, I strongly recommend Richard Gerber's *Vibrational Medicine for the 21st Century* as *the* place to start.

One more point. As I know only too well, it is easy to indulge in complementary therapy overload. What we don't realize is that this can be counterproductive, and you can end up with your body not knowing which way, energetically, to turn next. This is why it's better to stay with one therapy at a time, and to make sure you tell your therapist what other therapies or remedies you've tried or are trying, however insignificant or benign they seem. I have promised myself to be better disciplined in future.

212

A note on healing therapies

The journey to recovery is a journey of choice.

— Dame Diana Mossop, Institute of Phytobiophysics

Healing is a word often used, yet little understood. It doesn't mean to get better from your complaint, but to *be* better in the broadest sense. For insomnia, which can sometimes be a manifestation of some deep malaise, healing therapies can open that particular Pandora's box better than others. However, as one healer pointed out to me, today there are so many variations that healing has become a kind of 'spiritual entertainment'. You can spend a lot of money flitting from one to the other. All the more reason to choose with care.

Hands-on healing has definitely helped me: on bad days it has picked me up from the floor; on good days it has enabled me to be 'clearer'. As my chiropractor (page 280) also points out, you can receive healing – but then what? Once energy moves, you need to move, too. That means action, changing your life so that the old patterns that have contributed to your malaise can be broken. Of course, having your energy shifted makes it easier for you to change, but at some point you have to take responsibility for finishing the job. In other words, it is not just your body that heals itself, you need to, as the Americans would say, get your ass in gear. In short, whether we accept it, or do anything about it, or not, the choices we make in life have a fundamental effect on our health and well-being – or, in our case, our inability to sleep. Which is why the quote from Dame Diana Mossop puts the finger on this healing lark nicely.

Complementary Therapies: Where to Start?

Here's a checklist of complementary therapies/techniques that can help alleviate insomnia/help you sleep better:

Acupuncture (page 220)
Aromatherapy (page 161)
Autogenics (page 156)

Iridology
Kinesiology
Light therapy

Ayurvedic medicine (page 215)
Bach Flower remedies (page 168)
Bio-energy medicine (page 229)
Biomagnetic therapy (page 231)
Bowen Technique
Buteko method

Chakra healing

Chiropractic
Colour therapy (page 171)
Cranial osteopathy
Crystal therapy
Dowsing
Herbalism
Homoeopathy (page 222)
Hydrotherapy/floatation

Hypnotherapy (page 224)
Indian head massage

Magnet therapy (page 171)
Massage (page 158)
Meditation (page 152)
Naturopathy
Phytobiophysics (page 167)
Progressive muscle relaxation
(page 155)
Psychotherapy/Transpersonal
psychotherapy
Reflexology
Reiki
Sophrology
Sound therapy (page 170)
Spiritual healing
La Stone therapy
Tai chi (page 151)
Traditional Chinese Medicine
(page 218)
Yoga (page 148)
Zero-balance theory

What the experts say – complementary therapies and insomnia

Lots of the anti-stress therapies would help, e.g. aromatherapy, zero balancing, reflexology, hypnotherapy or cranial osteopathy, but only if you find a good therapist who knows what they are doing.

Nobody wants to be a guinea pig, so ask if the therapist you want to see has experience of treating your condition, where they trained, what accreditation or governing body they belong to and what their longer-term treatment regimen would be for you.

One of the very best treatments for insomnia is the Ayurvedic *shirodhara* where, after a soothing massage, you lie on the bed and have warm oil drizzled over your third eye for 40 minutes – but again, although this treatment has become popular in trendy London hotels, it is hard to find a good practitioner outside India.

— Susan Clark, *The Sunday Times*, 'What's the Alternative?' column

zzzz

Shirodhara may sound messy, but it's wonderful (see page 280).

Ayurvedic and Traditional Chinese Medicine

These are two of the great medical disciplines the world has to turn to, both far more ancient (and some say wiser) than Western medicine. As one practitioner qualified in both explains, Ayurvedic and Traditional Chinese Medicine are different cultural expressions of essentially the same kind of approach: holistic, energetically-based disciplines which marry the energetic qualities of nature with the energetic qualities of the person.

Both systems assess the constitution – physical and energetic – of the person, take the healing effect of diet very seriously, and make full use of herbal remedies. Traditional Chinese Medicine is very precise and clinically accurate; Ayurveda has more of an emphasis on constitutional types and lifestyles. Both systems involve the client in taking personal responsibility for their health. As far as insomnia and poor sleep are concerned, both belong to the 'A' Team. Both have their relaxation and spiritual counterparts in Yoga, Tai chi and Chi Kung. Illness is expressed not in terms of anatomy or physiology, but in terms of imbalance, and good health in terms of re-balancing and harmonizing the body/mind/spirit.

Ayurvedic medicine

Ayurvedic medicine and philosophy, 'the science of life', has been practised in India for over 4,000 years. It is founded on the belief that all life is a combination of the fundamental elements of nature: air, space, fire, water and earth. These combine to form three essential types or energies: air/ether (*Vata*), fire/water (*Pitta*) and water/earth (Kapha). Your fundamental constitution (*Dosha*) depends on which types are dominant; the subtle interplay of these three basic energies, combined with your genetic predisposition, are what makes you unique. Your *Dosha* qualities thus amount to your fingerprint. Doshas are both friend (when in balance) and foe (when out of balance), and shape your personality type as well as which health and illness traits you have a propensity for. Illness represents imbalances in your Dosha. Ayurvedic medicine uses diet and lifestyle to correct this.

Ayurveda marries your inner nature with Nature at large. Central to this is the notion of the seasons – something we forget these days, but which affects us far more than we realize. Doshic qualities shift and change with your life and the seasons, so you constantly need to be fine-tuning yourself. Ayurveda employs diet, detoxification, medicinal plants, massage, meditation, lifestyle activities and medicinal remedies specifically formulated for each Dosha, with the aim of restoring balance, the font of vitality and all well-being.

As well as taking medical details, determining a patient's Dosha and assessing his or her constitution are the first things Ayurvedic practitioners do.

Like Chinese medicine, Ayurveda has much to commend it. It forces you to look at your lifestyle in a different way. *The Book of Ayurveda, a Guide to Personal Well-being*, is one of the best places to start. The specialist Ayurvedic supplier, Pukka Herbs, website offers another excellent introduction and also lists Ayurvedic practitioners, includes a questionnaire to assess your own Dosha, lifestyle recommendations for your Dosha, and seasonal tips. Fascinating stuff!

What the experts say – Ayurveda and insomnia

Insomnia is a typical Vata complaint. The pressures of modern life are also Vata-aggravating (excess travelling, stimulation and a fast pace of life), so it's also a common one. Any one of the three constitutions can develop insomnia. Vata types have the most common tendency; Pitta types can also develop insomnia, but are more difficult to treat as anxiety and heat are often combined; it is less common among Kapha types.

The primary Ayurvedic treatment is to bring Vata back into balance. I would tackle diet and lifestyle first, and put the patient on an anti-Vata diet. This means eliminating obvious stimulants like caffeine, and avoiding any foods that are cold, dry or light, such as salads, popcorn and beans, and substituting these with grounding, heavy and warming foods. Oats are perfect as they are warming and help to nourish the nervous system. Other suitable foods are milk, nutmeg, quinoa and rice. I would also probably prescribe sedative herbs, such as Indian valerian to relieve the acute symptoms, and herbs to help restore the balance of the constitution in the long term, such as ashwangandha. I would recommend a warm sesame oil foot massage before going to bed, which specifically draws Vata down. Another crucial element of treatment is to encourage the patient to take up a soothing style of yoga and to start to use breathing practices in their daily programme.

Success depends on patient compliance – which is not always easy – and on what other issues need to be tackled. Insomnia is a classic out-of-balance condition. We all have our threshold, it just depends how far over the threshold we have gone. Ayurveda is a whole-life discipline and will ask you to make those changes if you want to be well again. For this reason I usually recommend another practitioner, e.g. a counsellor, as necessary, so the patient gets the best he/she deserves.

— Sebastian Pole, Ayurvedic and Chinese herbalist

Ayurveda and sleep

Ayurveda teaches that sleep is the wet nurse of the world; that to sleep on your right side is the most relaxing, the left is best for digestion, the back is very disturbing for Vata types and the stomach is no good for anyone. Ayurveda and Feng Shui have different ideas on where your head should be (which is confusing, I know, but I guess you'll have to investigate for yourself which is best for you). Ayurvedic teaching says that sleeping with the crown of your head in the East and feet towards the West promotes meditative sleep; head to the South promotes health; head to the North draws energy out of the body; head to the West encourages disturbing dreams. It also recommends that you always wash your face, hands and feet, massage your feet with oil (sesame is best) and meditate for a few moments before you go to bed.

The Book of Ayurveda explains that evening is Kapha time. Kaphas usually sleep well; if they sleep too much, kapha increases and they can't get up. Vatas need plenty of rest to replenish their nervous system (no late nights or night shifts). Not being able to get to sleep and waking up frequently, especially in the early morning (2 a.m.–4 a.m.) indicates that Vata is too high. Pittas need less sleep than the other two, and usually wake up bright and ready to go. If you wake up around midnight this indicates that your Pitta is too high.

- Put all this lot together, and you get the following advice to help lull you towards sleep: Sitting up in bed, watch your breath, reflect on the day, and give thanks.
- Put the light out and get yourself into a comfy sleeping position.
- If you fidget, don't worry, it's just your excess Vata. Watch your breath, breathe gently and deeply, and imagine yourself fast asleep (again).
- If you wake in the night, repeat the process – even if you don't sleep, it will help ensure that your body is rested.

Vata Tips

Vata types (like me) are especially prone to insomnia. Three painless Ayurvedic suggestions are easy to build into your life:

1. Make a flask of hot water flavoured with fresh ginger root and/or lemon juice, and drink it through the day. Vatas need warming up to counteract all the air (kinetic) energy responsible for communication, nerve flow, and all forms of activity.
2. Have some hot milk with plenty of grated nutmeg at bedtime. If you are allergic to cow's milk, substitute organic almond, rice, oat or soya milk.
3. Take ashwangandha, available as a tincture or herbal capsules, to help nourish your constitution and soothe frayed nerves. For more on ashwangandha, see page 131.

Traditional Chinese Medicine (TCM)

Traditional Chinese Medicine is as least as old as Ayurveda. It is an elegant, multi-layered medicine which offers a unique understanding of the human body, emotions and spirit. In essence, it's about the interplay of the female and male forces, yin and yang, and how these react with the elements that reside in each of us and all around us: wood, earth, fire, metal, air and water, and with the corresponding emotions associated with each element; how all of these are expressed in the organs of the body, and how all of these change with the seasons. Over-layered on this is the all-embracing concept of *chi*, life-force, or vital energy – equivalent to *prana* in Ayurvedic philosophy – which gives the body the power to heal itself. In TCM,

z z z z

chi flows through the body in energy channels or meridians. These run from top to toe and vice versa, act like an 'energy bloodstream' (and look that way, too, when represented diagrammatically), and are accessed through a series of acupuncture points (where acupuncture needles are inserted) or acupressure points (the same points, but where manual pressure with the thumb or finger is applied – for examples, see page 221).

To a Westerner's ears, though simple in concept, in practice TCM is quite complex.

Diagnostically, it is similarly eclectic. Tongue and organ pulse diagnosis – not to be confused with the blood pressure pulse – take the place of the GPs stethoscope. This is because, according to the principles of Eastern medicine, organs don't just perform a physical function but are fields of intelligence. They say something important about you, particularly your emotional intelligence. Acupuncture and herbal remedies and dietary regimes take the place of drugs. Indeed, the Chinese medical knowledge and understanding of food as medicine are unsurpassed.

Where does this leave insomnia? In China, considerable research has been done on the efficacy of acupuncture and Chinese herbal medicine in treating insomnia. In the US there are TCM practitioners who specialize in identifying which particular pattern of insomnia a patient has, and treating him or her accordingly. Internally, generally insomnia is a result of excess yang, itself a consequence of organ imbalance. The main organs involved are the heart, liver, gallbladder, spleen and kidneys. As Professor Chen (see page 283), known for her success in treating insomnia, explains:

It's a question of finding which organ(s) is the primary cause. An imbalance in the kidney (water) will automatically lead to an imbalance in the liver (fire); the two combined will cause yang to rise; this will express itself in the heart symptoms – for example, insomnia.

Imbalance of the heart means lack of joy, resentment, hatred (excess means too much fire or excitability); imbalance of the the liver means anger and frustration; of the spleen, worry; of the kidneys, fear and depression. Don't forget, either, that your adrenals sit on top of your kidneys, and your heart is where *shen* or 'spirit' resides. When *shen* is all over the place, so is your mind. No wonder we can't sleep.

Curing Insomnia Naturally with Chinese Medicine, by Bob Flaw (Blue Poppy Press Inc.) may be one book you'll find you can't resist.

Acupuncture

Acupuncture is the medicine of life-force, a technique to balance yin and yang. It achieves this by using very fine tiny sterilized needles or 'points' to access *chi* (life-force) via specific meridian points, in order to unblock the blockages responsible for illness, and to rebalance *chi*.

Recent research suggests that acupuncture can benefit insomnia, especially in re-establishing disturbed sleep–wake cycles. These days, too, you can measure acupuncture points electronically, and use machines instead of needles (see bio-energetic medicine, page 229).

As acupuncturists will confirm, insomnia often expresses itself as heart fire; the remedy is to 'calm the mind and smooth the chi in the blood'. Though you could go to 20 different acupuncturists and they might all give you slightly different treatments, the diagnostic approach outined above will be the same. Speak to the helpline *Sleep Matters* (page 191) and they will also tell you that people often have the most success in improving their sleep through acupuncture. If your insomnia is recent, before it gets a hold, acupuncture should be high on your list of possible treatments.

Usually an acupuncturist would expect to see a patient once a week for up to six weeks, and longer if the condition has persisted over many years (a basic rule of thumb is one week's treatment for every year you've been suffering from a complaint). You may also be prescribed Chinese herbs. If the diagnosis is correct, improvement generally happens soon.

Acupuncture can sound frightening, but isn't in the slightest. The needles are tiny – the only time you feel them, or they cause a bit of discomfort, is when there is a severe imbalance. They are not left in long. I have had needles in just about every bit of me, from my head to my toes, and there have been times when my acupuncturist has literally got me back on my feet. In my experience, too, acupuncturists are gentle, caring souls. In retrospect I should have focused on it for my insomnia more. As usual, I was trying all and sundry, and all at once.

Self-help: Acupressure points to help alleviate insomnia

Heart 7

The major acupressure point to calm the over-active, worried mind (and alleviate insomnia). It's located on the corner of the inside of the wrist, palm-side up, down from your little finger, on the crease, in a little dent by the wrist bone. Cupping your wrist with one hand and pressing or massaging this point gently for one minute, using your thumb, helps to induce calm. You can also now buy cheap self-adhesive plastic 'sleep well' cones that you stick on your wrist overnight and which do the job for you, which I've tried, though acupuncturists I've consulted doubt their effectiveness. I agree.

Heart 9

This also calms excess heat, and controls the thyroid. It's located at the end of the little finger, on the outside edge by the nail bed. Again, press or rub gently for one minute.

To help promote restful sleep, Dr Jennifer Harper (www.jenniferharper.com) in her excellent book *Nine Ways to Body Wisdom*, suggests holding the heart points in a warm bath containing Dead Sea Salts, which are rich in calming magnesium, potassium and calcium – a tip I follow. She also recommends specific essential oils to add to your bath: lavender and palmarosa.

Pericardium or 'Heart Protector'

This is the other important meridian associated with insomnia. Its function is to prevent anything harmful from reaching the heart.

Pericardium 6

This is the 'spirit point', located on the inside of the forearm, $2^1/2$ finger-widths from the wrist crease. It enhances our ability to relate to ourselves, our partners and the outside world, and helps support frazzled emotions. Hold for one minute to relieve anxieties, especially abut relationships.

Pericardium 7

This is located on the inside of the wrist, on the midpoint of the crease. It is another powerful supporting aid to relationship problems and to calm the spirit. Hold for one minute.

According to Dr Jennifer Harper, men often respond better to Heart Point 7, women to Pericardium 7. Working on them both simultaneously (easily done) enhances the beneficial results.

These points are comforting to know about and to have in your tool box. I like using them during the night, in the bath, or for those times when I'm feeling especially troubled. Read *Liberation* by the Barefoot Doctor, too, where you will learn more about all of this (and your organs), and much more besides.

Homoeopathy

Homoeopathy is the most beautiful and gentle 'honouring' therapy there is, the one we all want to work because it seems so right and natural. A homoeopath will aim to treat the underlying cause of your insomnia, be it physical, mental or emotional, and prepare a remedy specifically for you, taken either as tiny sublingual pilules or liquid drops.

Homoeopathy stimulates the healing power within you. Its founding principle, 'like cures like,' is that if a substance can trigger symptoms, a minute dose of the same substance will encourage the body to fight and overcome it naturally: think of it as a holistic vaccination.

Homoeopathic remedies are all animal-, mineral- or vegetable-based, and are so dilute that only the vibrational energy or 'memory' of the original substance remains – yet this can be remarkably powerful. The remedies are safe, non-addictive and can be used by anyone, including babies.

Two-and-a-half years into chronic insomnia, I found a remarkable homoeopath (Nicky Pool – she's a star!) and believe utterly that her help significantly enabled me to tackle insomnia from the inside out. Do not necessarily expect an easy ride, however. One tiny pill was all I got, but it was enough to send my not very good sleep pattern haywire for a short time, as I literally relived all my major symptoms, including the fears and anxiety of not being able to sleep, and much else besides. A temporary worsening of symptoms is common and to be expected – music to a homoeopath's ears, as it shows the remedy is working. Homoeopathic remedies may also induce feelings of well-being and optimism. What you can be sure of is that the reaction is unique to you, and is therapeutically beneficent.

With homoeopathy, little is everything. The more chronic the complaint, the less of a remedy you need to take. Unlike conventional drugs, you stop taking the remedy as soon as possible, and immediately you feel improvement. The remedy, incidentally, is coated on the *outside* of the tablet. This is why you need to be so careful not to handle them, but to transfer them under your tongue directly from the bottle, or use a clean spoon.

If you believe that your insomnia, like mine, is some kind of 'wake-up call', seeking help from a homoeopath is well worth a try. Just don't necessarily expect instant relief. You need to trust in the process – or, rather, the re-processing homoeopathy will kick into play. As Tony Pinkus (see page 224) reminded me, too, have faith in yourself as well as in the homoeopath, as it is you who eventually will have to be your own cure. If you don't – or can't – it's probably better to go elsewhere.

Over-the-counter homoeopathic remedies

These are widely available, and many people, including Nick (see page 70), have found them helpful. Don't confuse them, however, with individual remedies formulated specifically for you. They don't pretend to cure, but offer general relief, especially for temporary insomnia or sleeping problems due to stress. Because of the nature of homoeopathy, they will be a better 'fit' and therefore help or work better for some people than others. They relax the mind, reducing the chatter and thus helping sleep come more easily. The ingredients in homoeopathic insomnia tablets follow typical formulations, such as kali brom, coffee, passiflora, avena sativa, alfalfa and valerian.

What the experts say – homoeopathy and insomnia

Homoeopathy is about finding a match at a particular moment in your life. Temporary bouts of not sleeping are part and parcel of life, but in my experience chronic insomnia is almost inevitably about fears and not being able to face up to or deal with crises in your life, or about yourself. The insomnia stops you from sleeping and therefore dreaming, which is where hopes and fears are played out, and forces you back into a situation you don't consciously want to accept but subconsciously know you need to.

Most people expect an instant physical benefit from homoeopathy, but with conditions like insomnia I believe its role is more akin to psychotherapy than conventional medicine. The right remedy can produce the same shift that it takes several years of psychotherapy to make – and it's that shift which unblocks the stoppage and allows you to move to a healthier position.

Most people don't want to or aren't able to accept that their insomnia is part and parcel of who they are, nor do they want to confront this, but desperately need help, so seek remedies to help them sleep instead. I began my career as a pharmacist and saw people on this conveyor belt of pills. It's the socially acceptable solution to treat symptoms and contain illness that way, but it doesn't do anything for the real cause.

In the final analysis, there is only one person who keeps you awake with insomnia and that's yourSELF. When people tell me they are afraid, or say 'I can't' (which usually means the same thing), I remind them of the acronym FEAR: 'false evidence appearing as real'. You need to accept your fear before you can move on. Allow yourself to feel the fears that are keeping you awake. Then, without resisting, feel the fear while asking for that fear to be accepted as part of you. Thinking about them is not real, though we all fall into the trap of believing the opposite. More importantly, thinking causes us to separate rather than integrate our fears. If you feel them, you will allow yourself to give yourself space to heal. Homoeopathy will help create that space.

– Tony Pinkus, director and chief pharmacist,
Ainsworths homoeopathic pharmacy

z z z z

Hypnotherapy

Hypnotherapy has a 200-year-old pedigree and proven track record. It also requires no effort on your part, so is an attractive option for desperate insomniacs or anyone consistently having trouble sleeping.

Everyone's susceptibility to being hypnotized is different (some of us are more resistant than others), and 100 per cent success cannot be guaranteed – though, as with all matters of the mind, your belief system and attitude play a large part in its effectiveness.

Hypnosis is not being put to sleep or in a trance, or made to do funny things like being a chicken, but a state of heightened awareness, induced through deep relaxation. What it does is talk directly to your subconscious, replacing old, unwanted patterns of behaviour, such as smoking, with new beneficial suggestions, such as not wanting to smoke. To do this the hypnotherapist needs to, as it were, tranquillize your conscious mind so it sits there as a silent observer, allowing your subconscious to come forward.

As Dr Alastair Dobbin, a practising GP and hypnotherapist, explains, insomnia or sleeping problems can sometimes be the easiest complaints for hypnotherapists to deal with. The ability to sleep is natural – our subconscious understands how to sleep, even if we don't. Here, it's primarily a question of clearing the decks or, in chronic cases, finding the 'virus' corrupting your 'mental hardware'.

A hypnotherapist will usually access your subconscious memory files to find out what triggered off your insomnia, hypnotize you directly to rectify this, and perhaps also give you an individually-scripted tape. Pre-recorded tapes will lull you into deep relaxation and then give you positive suggestions for re-establishing your natural ability to sleep. You can also learn to hypnotize yourself.

I think hypnotherapy is definitely worth a try, though don't necessarily expect a quick fix, especially if your insomnia is the tip of a complicated iceberg. Here, you may need a step-by-step approach. As someone who is not good with exotic white beaches fringed with palm trees, whispering brooks or any other forms of visualization, I approached hypnotherapy with some cynicism, which, as it happened, turned out to be totally unfounded. Being hypnotized was nothing like I'd imagined, either. It is nothing to be concerned about, and you really are 'all there'. It didn't provide a cure at the time (I was been advised to wait until I'd finished this book, so my mind couldn't sabotage the treatment), but by the time you read this book, I hope to be well and truly sorted.

What the experts say – hypnosis and insomnia

Hypnosis is one of the most valuable treatments for all kinds of emotional and mental ailments, including insomnia. Suggestion hypnosis, including tapes and self-hypnosis, have about a 30 per cent success rate, I find. It is particularly useful for patients with transient or straightforward insomnia. If insomnia is chronic, however, or it has persisted for years, it is invariably due to a trauma at some time in the patient's life. This can hinge on something as simple as a word, thought, or vision implanted at the time of the traumatic event. Such patients need regression therapy. The hypnotist has to isolate the time when the trauma became embedded into the subconscious – usually in childhood – and remove it. It's like having a rogue file in your subconscious which gets activated at a later date. The hypnotherapist's job is to find the virus and reprogramme the file. This will usually take 3–5 sessions and works in 80–90 per cent of cases. It is dependent on the practitioner's skill at regression and/or the client's subconscious, which sabotage the new messages because of a secondary motive: at some level the patient isn't ready, for whatever reason, to be healed. That said, just about all of my insomniac patients over the last 20 years have been cured, and stay cured, with this method.

Hypnosis can improve the quality of sleep for many people, not just those with sleep problems. My work involves running two-day self-hypnosis courses for companies and organizations to help employees de-stress their lives. As a result, about 75 per cent report better sleep and increased productivity. Recent scientific studies have confirmed this, and have shown that hypnosis improves the passage of blood to the brain, as well as improving immune function.

– Valerie Austin, Harley Street consultant hypnotherapist and author of *Self-hypnosis*

Hypnotherapy tapes

These follow similar patterns, but have individualized scripts. They all use words like 'deep' and 'relax', make use of standard tried-and-tested ways to induce you into deep relaxation (such as imagining going down in a lift), contain instructions on how to come out of the hypnosis, use positive affirmations about loving yourself or something similar – and then get down to the business of making you believe you can sleep. You can play them as often as you like, and at any time – they work better when you're not paying attention, but I find bedtime and during the lonely hours especially useful. In a short time they become like a dummy, and will often put you to sleep after the first few phrases. This has the double bonus that the tape will also be more effective because your subconscious has a clear run.

Note that this doesn't always happen: you will spend a lot of time just listening, but – and it's an important but – you do get the benefit of training yourself to relax deeply, which is an immediate stress-reliever and helps make up for your lack of sleep.

A couple of practical thoughts

1. The most infuriating thing about tapes is usually the tape-recorder you use. Many whir, and click loudly when the tape has finished. This can wake you up, or is a distraction when you're trying to listen and be peaceful. Check this before you buy or use a tape machine or CD player. A CD player with a replay facility is really what you want for subliminal messages.
2. Battery recorders eat batteries; if you have one, rewind the tapes on a tape machine plugged into the mains.

'Pillow Talk' headphones, made by Roberts, work well.

Subliminal Tapes and CDs

Subliminal recordings are the hypnotherapy equivalent to subliminal advertising, except they are for your good. In the first ones I tried (Pilgrim Tapes, page 253), the speech is speeded up so it sounds like high-pitched gibberish, which you then turn down until it is no longer audible. Often a script is hidden underneath the one you are actively listening to. They are brilliant because the suggestions go directly to your subconscious. Please note that these will also 'cure' anyone else who happens to be within earshot, if they so need or desire – which can be handy. These types of tapes and CDs are an act of faith, maybe, but testimonials abound to their efficacy.

Brainwashing or cure?

Therapists get very agitated if you point out that subliminal suggestions are the same as brainwashing. The difference is that brainwashing is covert: you haven't a clue what's going on, what is being said, or what it's for; nor have you chosen to listen to them.

InnerTalkUK®

This company produce cutting-edge subliminal life-changing/ -enhancing CDs, developed by American research scientist Eldon Taylor and formulated using the Whole Brain® or Progressive Awareness Research (PAR), whereby both sides of the brain are addressed with slightly different messages (in a way each side can accept best).

The CDs are designed to bypass your conscious mind entirely and reprogramme your subconscious mind to change your current behaviour for the better. The subliminal positive affirmations are silently buried in sublimely soothing music or sounds of the ocean. The more you play them, the faster the results; what I do is to turn them down to a whisper, and let them play all night; during the day I play them as background while I'm working.

Their insomnia tape is called 'Sleep Soundly'. The script contains two sorts of affirmations: one about sleep and another about feeling good about yourself and life. Most people, myself included, prefer the sounds of the ocean at night instead of music, which are themselves soporific (see page 170). Though I didn't expect to, I find it beautifully soothing. They also offer a free 'Forgiveness' CD, which you might want to consider.

You can expect results within three weeks. With insomnia it's not uncommon to have a rapid improvement at first, then a lapse – explained as your subconscious making its last stand at sabotaging or resisting before taking on board the new script fully. This is what happened to me: a miracle cure for five days, then back to square one. Persevere. If you don't see any improvement at all, you may

z z z z

need to dig deeper and treat that first. This is common among men, for whom stress issues are often being masked by their insomnia.

The recordings are carefully scripted to be typical. They suit most people, most of the time. For this reason they do not claim to cure insomnia, nor to be a substitute for medical treatment, but they are mightily useful to have in your self-care kit. I've become a fan. For more, see www.innertalk.co.uk or their American research site: www.progressiveawareness.org. Be warned: you could get addicted, especially when you read the list of what they have to offer. All of a sudden getting the perfect you and the perfect life won't seem so difficult at all.

Bio-energy medicine

Energy medicine takes many forms, from modern laser therapy to the latest sound–colour chromoson therapy, developed by a Belgian scientific-spiritual group, Les Sciences Naturelles. Over the last 50 years, notably in Germany and Russia, a different kind of energy medicine has emerged, one that employs sophisticated electro-diagnoses with specially designed equipment to bio-assay exactly what's happening to your electro-conductivity or energy fields, variously known as bio-energy, bio-resonance or bio-functioning medicine. It's used extensively to monitor the effects of space travel on Russian cosmonauts. It's precise, objective but also holistic (for *chi,* just think electro-energetic fields of the body instead), as are the practitioners who use it.

The tests involved are painless and very simple, and take only a few minutes to complete. Seeing your brain waves come up on a computer screen is revealing, to say the least.

The use of acupuncture is fundamental to bio-energy medicine, though practitioners don't use needles but lasers or weak microwave signals. Treatment often includes homoeopathic, nutritional or herbal remedies, and may include wiring you up to get re-balanced – though be wary of practitioners who use only machines to cure you; the machine's role should be primarily diagnostic.

For insomnia, bio-energy medicine can be very helpful; if the root cause is microtoxicity in the brain, for example, this is one technique

z z z z

that should winkle it out. This approach should also be able to assess whether your insomnia is primarily psycho-somatic or somato-psychic.

Bio-energy medicine is well established in Europe and the US, but there are only a handful of specialists in the UK; Thomas Manifold-Marshall (see below) and Anthony Scott-Morley (page 265) are two of the most experienced. Both stress that they do not treat conditions but people; and that for chronic complaints you need to find all the factors, visible and hidden, and treat them in the right order.

My case

My brain-frequency analysis indicated an imbalance of my hypothalamus–pituitary function, resulting in low hormonal levels. The meridian-system analysis showed energy levels to be reasonable, except for three rather nasty dips – Liver, Kidneys and Spleen, the three yin meridians most associated with hormone imbalance. Stress was a persistant factor in both the brain frequency and body scan (decoder demograph). A heavy-duty course of Chinese herbal formulas followed, addressing hormonal imbalance, sleep, and blood deficiency. Within a short time I felt calmer and generally more peaceful; though still erratic, my sleep improved. A follow-up scan two months later revealed that my liver and kidney function were much improved; my spleen was not, and there was still a question mark over my blood deficiencies. Whoever said getting cured was easy?

What the experts say – bio-energy medicine and insomnia

For an initial consultation at my clinic I use three bio-diagnostic tests. The first is measurement of the Chinese meridian system using the advanced microprocessor probe developed by the Russians to monitor cosmonauts; the second, especially important in sleep disorders, [is] a brain-frequency analysis which measures Delta, Theta, Alpha and Beta frequencies – it's like scanning FM on the radio 10 times and mapping out areas of weak signals; the third is the Decoder Dermograph – an energetic scan of seven sections of the body taken from electrodes connected between head, hands and feet. The result is a very accurate snapshot of where the patient is bio-energetically, both physically and psychologically. The discrepancies/abnormalities/imbalances detected in the cross-referencing of all three tests relate to whole functioning of the patient.

z z z z

Brain-frequency analysis, for example, plays an essential role in all major functions. Hormonal control is associated with Theta frequencies; memory and concentration and deep sleep with Delta frequencies; while Beta frequencies are associated with regulation through the Pituitary/Hypothalamus/Adrenal axis, and therefore sugar, sleep and thermostat control. It is often found that people who are wide awake at 3 a.m., for example, have had a blood sugar dip, which causes an adrenal surge in order to raise the sugar levels, resulting in a form of insomnia where the patient is 'wide awake' and could do a week's housework there and then. On the Decoder body scan, disturbances or abnormal energetic levels may be associated with sleep problems, where there is evidence of electrical disturbances due to the influence of computer VDUs and digital alarm clocks, which can build up electrical currents with tooth amalgams. Disturbances may also indicate neck or jaw subluxations affecting blood and cerebral spinal fluid flow.

All complementary practitioners understand that the causes of chronic insomnia are multi-dimensional. If from my overall evaluation of a patient I judge that emotional or psychological factors predominate, then, coupled with appropriate homoeopathic and herbal prescriptions, I will also recommend NLP [neuro-linguistic programming] therapy, as I find this very effective in helping people to take their current dilemmas in hand and give them the tools that can help them through.

– Thomas Marshall-Manifold DC, Lic.Ac., Lic.O.H.M, D.Sc.,
Wimbledon Clinic of Natural Medicine, London

Biomagnetic therapy

This is completely different from either bio-energy medicine or the use of fixed high-strength magnetic aids such as pillow pads (page 172). It's a specialized, precise acupuncture treatment developed by Dr Osamu Itoh in the 1970s, which utilizes weak dot magnets to stimulate the master points of the Eight Extra-ordinary acupuncture meridians to enable faster and more effective rebalancing of energy channels and structural distortions. It's used for a variety of complaints, including stress and sleeping problems. The treatment is simple, painless, and you should expect noticeable improvement in about three sessions.

Conclusion

Like any insomniac, I fervently hoped I would have my eureka moment and find my 'cure' while writing this book. That I hadn't by the time the manuscript was handed in was a bitter disappointment, but I consoled myself that I was at least in the same boat as my readers. But I have reached some conclusions:

For insomniacs

- Each person's insomnia is unique to him or her.
- Only we can truly cure ourselves.
- You need to acknowledge and 'own' your insomnia. There's no point blaming somebody else or expecting someone or something to do all the work for you.
- Insomnia needs a multi-disciplinary approach – that is, you need your own personalized tool kit of things that help *you*.
- Variety is key. If one technique/remedy is no longer helping, move on. Don't get bored or give up the search for a solution(s) for you.
- Learn to be kind to yourself. It's the quickest way to be kind to everyone else, too.
- Recognize that managing your sleep is a trade-off. Sometimes you will trade life for sleep. This means you will choose to watch a late-night movie, go out and enjoy yourself, and do all the other things that 'normal' people do. Your sleep will probably suffer that night; don't fret about it. It's your choice. Living

the life of a mole is fine in theory, but we all need a break now and then.
- Many wise words and good advice have been written about insomnia and poor sleep. It's all valid, but don't expect it all to apply to you. Cherry pick. It'll make you feel much better.
- Insomnia is inevitably a journey of some kind; be prepared to adapt and change.
- Saying good-bye to insomnia is as big a lesson as the need to embrace it in the first place. The day will come when it will be time to put yourself back on the agenda, and to relegate sleep to the back-burner, where it belongs. Henceforth, ban the word 'insomnia' from your vocabulary.

For partners
- Insomnia is a miserable bedfellow which inevitably imposes strains on a relationship.
- Don't take it personally; become a temporary saint and understand that whatever you may think privately, the insomniac knows best. That, and hugs, help most of all.
- Above all, don't let your own sleep suffer. Two miserable sleep-deprived people are a recipe for disaster.

For everyone else
- If your insomnia or poor sleep is temporary, *please* don't go into obsessional overdrive. It happens to everyone. But do nip it in the bud *now*.
- If you are reading this book because you want to sleep better, well done! Sleep is a beautiful and precious gift. We should all nurture it and care for it as tenderly as we can.
- Spread the word, and make sure your family and friends get streetwise about good sleep, too.

Good luck, best wishes, and very, very sweet dreams.

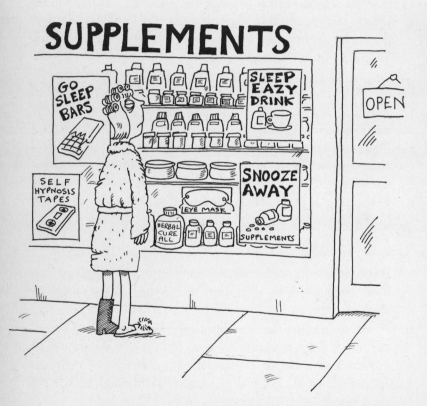

PART 4

Sleeping directory and resources

Website directory

Internet chat forums

Internet chat forums are the most informal way to get help, or share your difficulties with someone who understands. They offer self-help and a chance for you not to feel so isolated. Two things quickly become clear: there are a lot of insomnia buffs out there who know an awful lot about their condition, so good advice and matters of interest are there to be had, if you have the time and the stamina, or just love the web. Secondly, you will read some unbelievably harrowing tales which will make your own insomnia seem trivial by comparison – which can be good therapy in itself. Inevitably, too, there is an awful lot of chit-chat, not to mention night-owls using potentially good-sounding chat forum sites as general gossip sites. Four genuine ones are:

www.circlecity.co.uk/sleepdesk

The Circle City Communities website. The only UK-based chat forum we've found. Its sleep desk section is devoted to insomnia and other sleep disorders and has its own message board for questions and interactive chat, advice, etc. Simple, easy to use and read, and has the virtue of being refreshingly short and basic.

www.insomniacure.com/pillowtalk.html

Exemplary dedicated, serious insomnia chat forum, run by American author and professional insomniac John Weidman. For more on this remarkable website, see page 241.

www.sleepnet.com

Another dedicated popular American sleep forum. If you are plucking up courage to sleep in the spare room away from a snoring partner, read Hope Star's story and be encouraged it can work out OK. For more on this, see page 241.

www.talkaboutsleep.com

A new American sleep website with its own live chat with sleep experts, and message board.

www.remedyfind.com

Just occasionally, the web comes up trumps. This American website has a sleep disorder section which focuses on insomnia. It gives info on a wide range of treatments including various sleeping pills, herbal sleep aids, relaxation techniques, etc., and ratings from insomniacs who've used them. You can also sign up for a regular free e-mail newsletter which includes personal stories and links to latest research. Useful as a snapshot on what's out there to help; especially useful if you want to find out more about prescription drugs and their brand names.

For other self-help advice services, see page 191.

Sleep websites

Want to be your own sleep expert? There is enough information on the web about sleep, sleep disorders and insomnia to keep you awake for ever. To make matters even more daunting, there are several excellent websites with fabulous links, chat rooms, message boards, sleep forums and all the rest of it.

z z z z

Here is a brief selection of what you can expect. You will not thank me for including more – this lot is more than enough for even the most ardent insomniac.

UK Websites

www.sleepspecialist.co.uk

New website set up by Professor Idzikowski, who runs The Sleep Assessment and Advisory Service (see page 191). Still being completed at time of going to press, but likely to be one of the best UK sleep websites.

www.neuronic.com

Professor Idzikowski's original website. They don't come much better or more inclusive than this. Includes its own web guide to insomnia, consumer sleep disorders directory (sleep aid products galore), alternative therapies, and lectures. Links to all his activities including the Sleep Assessment and Advisory Service, and www.thepuresleep.com (page 260).

http/Sleep.lboro.ac.uk

No www prefix required. Website of Loughborough Sleep Disorder Centre, one of the UK's foremost sleep research centres. Includes general articles by Professor Horne, which are worth reading.

www.londonsleepcentre.co.uk

Excellent website for the recently opened London Sleep Centre in Harley Street.

www.sleeping.org

Website for The British Sleep Society, the medical professional body promoting good sleep. If you want to see who's who in the British sleep world, or see the kind of research questions that occupy sleep scientists, this is the place to look. For details of how to obtain their UK Sleep Provider list, see page 268.

www.sleepcouncil.com

Sleep Council website, funded by the bed industry. Good info on beds and how to find the right one for you; plus details of insomnia helpline.

Finally, in need of a bit of diversion? Two product-orientated websites that will offer you cures galore are:

www.bestenginesearch.co.uk – lists the UK's 'Top Ten' insomnia websites, who really want you to know about them, with links. Includes *Which?* on line, websites offering melatonin, deep sleep hypnosis tapes, etc.

www.searchy.co.uk – same thing and yet more search links to do with insomnia.

US Websites

Sleep-deprivation is big business in the US – 20 million Americans suffer from insomnia – with sleep websites to match, run primarily by private companies and charitable institutions who specialize in sleep health care. Generally excellent, virtually all contain information over-load, and it's a question of navigating your way through to find the nuggets that may help you. For sleep-deprivation buffs only. If you only want to read one, try
www.americaninsomniaorganization.org

www.sleepfoundation.org

The granddaddy of them all and website of America's National Sleep Foundation (NSS), founded in 1990. Pioneering sleep scientist William C Dement is a former president. First-rate information, and lots of it! Impressive (largely academic) links section, plus helpful advice and tips, including a caffeine-calculator so you can work out your own caffeine overload.

z z z z

www.aasmnet.org

America's foremost professional membership organization, dedicated to the advancement of sleep and related research. Includes country-wide search for local AASM – accredited centres and laboratories.

www.sleepmed.com

Website of Sleep Medicine Associates of Texas Inc, largest private sleep centre and laboratory, with over 30 years experience. Masses of information, most found under 'Maximizing the quality of your sleep', much familiar/technical but useful advice and tips scattered throughout. Easy-to-use website. Limited usefulness for UK readers.

www.sleepnet.com

Or 'everything you ever wanted to know about sleep but were too tired to ask'. Impressively good zany educational website, one of my favourites, run by an indefatigable sleep scientist called Sandeman. Clear information, arranged in bite-sized bits, which manages to be both informative and entertaining, plus add-ons such as a sleep questionnaire to work out your own sleep status. Popular public sleep forum (see page 238). Awesome world-wide links section, which includes site reviews and ratings.

www.americaninsomniaassociation.org

The one website I wish I had found earlier. Website for the American Insomnia Association (see page 284). The most comprehensive and pithy account you will find about insomnia and how to deal with it.

www.insomniacure.com

Insomniac's heaven (or hell). Amazing website of America's most famous 'professional insomniac', John Weidman, author of *Desperately Seeking Snoozin'*, dedicated to insomnia, with excellent info, tasters from his book, and chat forum (see page 238). Formidably impressive links section, with helpful guidelines and brief descriptions.

z z z z

www.prescriptionforsleep.com

Website for Prescription for Sleep, a company who run sleep courses addressing sleep deprivation in the workplace and in schools. Excellent website, clearly presented with good information and advice, no waffle.

www.deepsoundsleep.com

Website for 'Deep Sound Sleep' and other sleep-promoting/insomnia-solving guided meditation tapes, produced by well-known American hypnotherapist and Soulologist Michaiel Patrick Bovenes. Useful 'alternative' website for tackling insomnia from the 'inside out'.

www.well-connected.com

The other website I wish I had found earlier. Another first-class comprehensive account of insomnia and what to do about it, written by experienced medical writers. Especially useful for where to get help for American readers; the portal you need is: http://wellness.ucdavis.edu/medical_conditions_az/insomnia27.html

www.talkaboutsleep.com

Latest grassroots website, founded by a sleep patient and doctor, aimed at both the public and the medical community, dedicated to disseminating information about sleep and sleep disorders including insomnia, and providing advice and support to sufferers. Includes live chat rooms, message board and the Insomnia Corner, which includes articles by Dr Gregg Jacob, author of *Say Goodnight to Insomnia*.

Finally,

www.angelfire.com/ca2/ericascourtyard/poetry.html

Something completely different. A poetry portal for insomniacs.

See also: internet chat forums and www.remedyfind.com, page 238.

z z z z

Sleep and insomnia books on-line

For the best selection of books on sleep and insomnia, visit www.amazon.com or www.amazon.co.uk; key in 'sleep' and 'insomnia'. But breathe very deeply first: www.amazon.com lists over 2,200 titles on sleep and 200 on insomnia; www.amazon.co.uk over 2,700 titles on sleep and 194 on insomnia. Each website also contains enough music CDs on the subject to keep you sleepy for ever. A more manageable list of books can be found on: www.neuronic.com/insomnia_bookstore.html

Websites at a glance

Here's a list of the websites mentioned in the text, in alphabetical order. On-line ordering for products is usually world-wide.

www.ainsworths.com

Website for renowned Ainsworths homoeopathy company. On-line pharmacy (over 3,000 remedies), magazine and links to homoeopathic sites.

www.aromatherapyassociates.com

Product website for Aromatherapy Associates. Wonderful list of products, difficult to resist, produced to very high standards. Includes list of UK outlets including SPNK shops.

www.a-t-c.org.uk

UK Aromatherapy Essential Oil Trade Association website. Useful information and web links, plus list of members and their websites. Leaflets available.

www.autogenic-therapy.co.uk

Website for British Autogenic Society; very good and very informative. Includes list of UK practitioners.

www.thebackcoach.com

Product website for neck and backstretchers, and book, *The Art of Backstretching* (recommended). Clear explanations, and on-line ordering.

www.biobrite.com

Light therapy and jet-lag info and products.

www.bioligo.com

Website for Swiss oligiotherapy specialists Laboratoires Biologico. In French and English; info on products and how trace minerals can help your health. On-line ordering.

www.bkwsu.com

Website for the Brahma Kumari World Spiritual University. Thoughtful website, easy to use. Includes details of their retreats in Rajasthan, New York, Italy, the UK and Australia. On-line shop.

www.blinds.co.uk

Specialist, value-for-money, made-to-measure blind company, including blackout blinds. Worth a look. On-line ordering.

www.blissfulmusic.com

Website for the Bliss music ensemble. The name describes their music perfectly. Includes events listing and on-line ordering for their CDs.

www.cmhmassage.co.uk

Website of international massage expert, Clare Maxwell-Hudson, and her London School of Massage. Details of courses and how to buy her books on-line.

www.dadamo.com

American blood type diet guru, Dr Peter J D'Adamo's Eat Right 4 You website. Huge. Learn all about blood type diets and check out which foods are right for your blood type.

z z z z

www.elemis.com

Elemis, lifestyle brand of high-quality aromatherapy skin and body-care products. Includes on-line spa shop and details of Elemis day spas in the UK and US.

www.floweressences.com™

One of the most impressive websites I've come across. If you want to find out about flower essences, and buy them, this is a must-visit site.

www.foodandmood.org

Website for the UK Food and Mood project, linking diet and mood and how to change your diet to improve your emotional/mental moods. Includes nutritional therapist search facility, and useful organizations/lab testing and nutritional supplements links.

www.fragrant.demon.co.uk

Global aromatherapy internet site. Info on aromatherapy and essential oils; world-wide lists of suppliers and practitioners.

www.gsdl.com

Great Smokies Diagnostic Laboratories website. This is where you get your hormones and biochemistry revealed. Worth a look.

www.healthplusweb.com

American internet alternative medicine resource site. Bursting with info; contains practitioner directory.

www.hearingprotection.co.uk

Website for Advanced Communication Solutions Ltd, who make Elacin sleepfits. Have agents world-wide. Fascinating info on understanding hearing, including safe listening times. Product info and on-line ordering.

www.herb.org

Seriously good website for American-based Herb Research Foundation, dedicated to the latest scientific research and comprehensive information about efficacy, health benefits and safety of herbs. Search facility. Publications and information packs available on line.

www.herbmed.org

Run by the Alternative Medicine Foundation Inc, another excellent dedicated information resource about the use of herbs for health for professionals, researchers and the general public. Search facility. Extensive links section to scientific data.

www.homeinonhealth.com

Website for Yorkwellbeing, supply diagnostic health check-kits, including for house dust mites and anti-allergy bedding. On-line ordering.

www.innertalk.com

Website of American parent company of Inner Talk subliminal self-development programmes.

www.innertalk.co.uk

Product website for Inner Talk UK subliminal tapes/CDs. Friendly site, useful info, on-line shopping, etc. Links to personal development/alternative health/spirituality sites.

www.jenniferharper.com

Website for naturopath, herbalist and TCM practitioner Dr Jennifer Harper. On-line ordering for her books and CDs.

www.jetlagsolutions.com

For serious travellers. Latest info and products on how to beat jet-lag.

www.kundaliniyoga.org

A rare gem, a website that really works. Fascinating and absorbing, beautifully executed, with on-line yoga training, complete with diagrams of yoga postures, simple and elegant explanations and wise thoughts. Learn all about the art and practice of kundalini yoga here. For help with sleep, go to lesson 16: Shabad Kriya: Bedtime Meditation.

z z z z

www.lightmask.com

English/American specialized medical light therapy company: explanatory info, scientific trials, testimonials and products (light mask and light boxes). Includes world-wide telephone/on-line ordering.

www.livingmovement.com

Website for Tai-chi expert and author, Angus Clark: includes details of his international courses.

www.luscher-color.com

Official (short) multilingual website for the Dr Max Luscher pyschophysical colour test, which measures the ability to withstand stress and communicate. Useful information about the test and Prof Max Luscher; on-line shop.

Plus: www.actualsystem.com

Provides computer DIY version of the Luscher colour test. Key in 'actual luscher' on home page.

www.moodcure.com

Website for nutritionist Dr Julia Ross, author of *Mood Cure*. Lots of info, details of her clinic and on-line shop. Buy Serotonin (5-HTP) and tryptophan here.

www.oligotherapy.co.uk

Website for UK Institute of Oligotherapy. E-mail consultations, on-line ordering and help to locate therapists (majority currently in SE England).

www.patrickholford.com

Optimum Nutrition guru Patrick Holford's website. Well worth a visit. Superb useful info section. On-line ordering for supplements, books, events, free e-mail newsletter and how to find an optimum nutritionist in the UK and US.

www.phytobiophysics.com

Institute of Phytobiophysics website. Learn all about phytobiophysics here. Includes on-line shop for flower remedies and details of UK and international practitioners, plus links.

www.pillowrx.com

American manufacturer (Mediflow) water pillow website. See what it is and how it works. On-line ordering.

www.progressiveawareness.org

Progressive Awareness Research Inc website. Information and research on subliminal technology.

www.pukkaherbs.com

Ayurvedic specialists and suppliers of premium organic and fairly traded Ayurvedic products, including remedies, teas and bodycare. Excellent website. On-line ordering.

www.quinessence.com

Website for Quinessence aromatherapy company, aromatherapy specialists for over 20 years. Includes excellent introduction to aromatherapy and essential oils; newsletter; on-line shop includes products, books and vaporizers.

www.richardlawrence.co.uk

Website of well-known mind/body/spirit teacher, author, broadcaster and lecturer. Also includes events and links to the Atherius Society, a non-profit-making healing organization. On-line ordering for his CDs and books.

www.riobeauty.com

Health/fitness/lifestyle product website. Includes aromatherapy/vaporizers and light masks. On-line ordering.

www.sacredsound.net

Website for Soundworks and the British Academy of Sound Therapy. Good background info on sound as healing, details of workshops, practitioner list and on-line 'retail therapy' shop for crystal and Tibetan bowls, accessories and Soundworks CDs.

www.sad.uk.com

Website for SAD. Lightbox company. Info on S.A.D., on-line sales.

www.smartlifenews.com

On-line American Smart Life News newsletter of CERI (Cognitive Enhancement Research Institute: **www.ceri.com**) dedicated to cutting-edge information on cognitive enhancement, health and longevity. Find out how to be smart; melatonin and 'smart hormones' here.

www.symbiosis-music.com

Website for Symbiosis music trio, specialists in relaxation music. On-line ordering for their CDs.

www.taichiuk.co.uk

Website of Zenon Wudang Tai Chi Chuan School, based in London and founded by Sifu Michael Jacques, British Tai Chi champion. Tai Chi, Kick Boxing, Chi Kung and Reiki. Good explanatory website, includes details of courses and classes throughout London.

www.theretreatcompany.com

Great website. Your chilled-out dreams start here. What's on and where to go around the world.

www.valerieaustin.com

Website for well-known Harley Street consultant hypnotherapist. Includes details of hypnotherapy in business, training, self-hypnosis and stress-reduction seminars, books, videos and tapes.

www.viniyoga.co.uk

Exemplary website, thoughtful and intelligent. Explanation of viniyoga, its roots, list of UK qualified and licensed practitioners and very good on-line yoga bookshop.

www.viridian-nutrition.com

Website for Viridian Nutrition Ltd. Friendly website, info on environment, products, store locator (UK, Holland, Spain and South Africa), links to several charity websites.

www.waterbed.co.uk

British Waterbed Company website. Includes useful FAQs and list of stockists.

www.whatreallyworks.co.uk

Health writer Susan Clark's ultimate insider's guide to what really works and lifestyle health website.

Products and services

Sleep-aid products and services

All products mentioned are available both in the UK and internationally; most offer 28-day money-back guarantee. Telephone numbers, where given, are for UK customers only.

Anti-allergy bedding

Yorkwellbeing

0800 074 6185
www.homeinonhealth.com
Part of Yorktest Group. Provide house dust mite home check-kits and range of anti-allergy bedding. On-line ordering.

Back and neck stretchers/magic pillows

Enanef Ltd

0700 222 5724
www.thebackcoach.com
e-mail: neil@thebackcoach.com
Run by back expert Neil Summers. Catalogue available.

Ged Codd (magic pillow)

01790 754444

Blackout blinds

Blinds.co.uk
0800 056 7446; 0207 375 1053
www.blinds.co.uk
e-mail: sales@blinds.co.uk

Earplugs

Elacin Sleepfits
Advanced Communication Systems Ltd (UK)
01582 767007
www.hearingprotection.co.uk
e-mail: info@hearingprotection.co.uk

Light boxes

SAD Lightbox Co Ltd
01494 484852/484851
www.sad.uk.com
Bright light box manufacturers, offer versatile range of boxes, each
operating at 2,500 and 10,000 lux, for home and office.

Light masks

The Dezac Group Ltd
Customer care line: 01242 702345 (not always manned)
www.riobeauty.com or www.lightmask.com

Light Therapy and Jetlag Products

On-line ordering from the US at:
www.biobrite.com
www.jetlagsolutions.com

Magnetic sleep aids

Norstar Biomagnetics Ltd
01635 588888
www.norstarbiomagnetics.com
e-mail: info@norstarbiomagnetics.com
UK leader in cutting-edge technology of therapeutic magnetic field therapy. Helpful customer service. Products include pillow and mattress pads. Also available: *The Magnetic Therapy Handbook* and *Magnetic Therapy* by founder Gloria Vergari.

Self-help CDs and cassette tapes

InnerTalkUK®
01628 898366
www.innertalk.co.uk
e-mail: info@innertalk.co.uk
People-friendly and happy to talk and give you advice on which programme they recommend for your circumstances. For the American parent company, see www.innertalk.com

Self-hypnosis cassette tapes

Pilgrim Tapes
01743 821270
Produced by Duncan McColl, hypnotherapist, behavioural consultant with 35 years experience. Cheap and very good.

Shiatsu massage table

Back in Action (UK)
www.backinaction.co.uk
e-mail: info@backinaction.co.uk
Distributors for the Shaitsu massage table, and sell waterbeds as well. Three Stores: London (tel: 0207 930 8309); Amersham (tel: 01494 434343); Marlow (01628 477177). Will ship world-wide.

Tension balls

People Tree
0845 450 4595; 0207 739 0660
www.ptree.co.uk
e-mail: sales@ptree.co.uk
Fair trade and eco-friendly fashion and handicrafts. Mail-order and on-line company. Their juggling balls, colourful hand-knitted hemp balls, made in Bangladesh, stuffed with flax seeds are cheap and good for squeezing hard. But mainly included because buying fair trade products (there are lots of nice things in the catalogue) helps make other people's lives better.

Nutritional/herbal supplements

All companies listed can ship world-wide. Telephone numbers given are for UK customers.

Higher Nature
0845 3300012 (order line)
0870 0664478 (nutritional advice service)
www.highernature.co.uk
Mail-order company. Ring for catalogue/newsletter. On-line shop. Supply 5-HTP and NeverSnore™.

The Nutri Centre
0207 436 5122
www.nutricentre.com
Retail store cum Aladdin's cave. UK's leading supplier of complementary medicines and nutritional supplements, and leading bookshop and information resource centre in complementary medicine. Stock over 20,000 books, including textbooks and journals (access to 70,000 titles); huge range (over 20,000) of nutritional supplements; music CDs/tapes, etc. Situated in the basement of the Hale Clinic. On-line shop. Mail world-wide. Supply Serotonin (5-HTP) and stabilium.

Solgar Vitamins Ltd

01442 890355
www.solgar.co.uk and www.solgar.com
e-mail:info@solgar.com
Well-known American nutritional supplement manufacturers, with respected reputation world-wide. Products generally available in health food stores, etc. Ring for nearest stockist; nutritional advice service also. For UK mail order, contact Boots Herbal Stores on 01782 617 463.

Viridian

01327 878050 (general/advice/nearest stockist)
www.viridian-nutrition.com
e-mail: info@viridian-nutrition.com
My favourite nutritional supplement company. Best Ethical Company award, 2003. Many organic products and 25 per cent of profits donated to charities. Phone for nearest stockist (over 500), or order on-line through Boots Herbal Stores at:
www.ethicalvitamins.co.uk.

Pukka Herbs

01608 659818
www.pukkaherbs.com
e-mail: sales@pukkaherbs.com
Ayurvedic specialists and pioneers in the organic Ayurvedic field. Comprehensive range of products available by mail-order or on-line, including herbs, capsules and essential oils, sourced from organic farms and fairly traded.
See also Stacktheme Ltd, page 268.

Serious sleep supplements

Melatonin

In the UK, available on prescription only. Available elsewhere as an over-the-counter aid for jet-lag. On the internet, available for personal shoppers from:

Natural Health Ministry (NHM Worldwide)

www.nhm.net
e-mail: jetlink@nhm.net
00353 1 4737881 (European call centre)
Approved by the Well Woman's Information Service. Supply Rest Assured melatonin sublingual tablets and Sound Sleep transdermal cream (blend of kava kava/melatonin and plant extracts); WGF serotonin support formula; WGF adrenal support formula; natural progesterone, other women's and men's health and anti-ageing supplements, and skin creams. 48-hour Jetlink service within Europe.

Biovea UK

www.biovea.co.uk
e-mail: support@biovea.co.uk
Supply a wide range of melatonin supplements; mood supplements including 5-HTP, SAM-E and Kavatrol (Kava-Kava); GABA; coral calcium; Thyroplex (thyroid supplement); vitamin and mineral supplements, women's and men's health and anti-ageing supplements.

Pricespower International Inc (US)

www.pricespower.com
US Orders (Toll Free): 00-1-800-927-9845
Weight-loss, diet aids and body-building supplements – and melatonin and 5-HTP, at competitive prices.

Vitacost (US)

www.vitacost.com
US Tel: 00-1-800-793-2601
Mail-order company, selling branded supplements at competitive prices. Can also be accessed through www.sleeping-tips.com.

Serotonin (5-HTP)

Available in the UK from Higher Nature and The Nutri Centre.
Available on the internet from:
www.biochemicals.com
www.biovea.co.uk

www.nhm.net
www.pricespower.com
www.vitacost.com

L-Tryptophan

In the UK, available on prescription only. On the internet, available for personal shoppers from:

The Mood Cure Nutrition Clinic (US)
www.moodcure.com

Bios Biochemicals (US)
www.biochemicals.com
Manufacturer of top-quality alternative practitioner supplements. Excellent information resource guide, and have a good article on sleep.

Products to reduce snoring

Two to get your partner to try:

Snoreeze
0800 096 1121 (UK freephone)
+ 44 207 731 7333 (outside UK)
www.snoreeze.com
A spray that lubricates and firms the muscles at the back of the throat (flabby muscles are the cause of snoring). On-line ordering. Money back if not satisfied.

NeverSnore™
Available from Higher Nature (page 254), and popular. The active ingredients are digestive enzymes that help break down mucus build-up at the back of the throat (another common cause of snoring). Eliminating dairy products also helps.

In the UK, Boots chemists also sell an oil-based lubricant, *Help Stop Snoring* Spray.

Anti-stress supplements

These include St John's Wort, GABA, rhodiola, kava-kava, ashwaganda and valerian.

All except kava-kava (see Biovea UK, page 256) are available from Solgar (page 255) and the Nutri Centre (page 254); most other companies listed offer a selection. Pukka Herbs (page 255) offer ashwaganda. St John's Wort and valerian are available from health stores, etc.

Herbal remedies

These are generally available from health stores. The companies listed above sell all or a selection, plus you might also like to try:

Hambleden Herbs

01823 401 205
www.hambledenherbs.co.uk
e-mail: info@hambledenherbs.co.uk
Award-winning specialist organic herb supplier (trade and retail) with a vast range of herbal remedies. On-line ordering.

Homoeopathic remedies

Ainsworths Homeopathic Pharmacy

0207 935 5330
www.ainsworths.com
Dedicated homoeopathic company, with over 20 years' experience, and respected reputation world-wide. Comprehensive selection of homoeopathic remedies (including sleep remedies) and Bach Flower remedies. On-line ordering.

Flower remedies

Flower Essence Pharmacy™ (US)

00-1-503-650-6015
www.floweressences.com
e-mail: info@floweressences.com
Remarkable company and flower essence pharmacy, stocking over 800 brands of flower essence remedies from Europe, Asia, North and South America, Australasia, Africa and the Pacific islands. One of the largest international distributors of vibrational flower remedies, plus Tibetan bowls, essential aromatherapy oils, etc. Excellent website contains full product information and description of each remedy sold, and all you want to know about flower remedies, including the latest research. On-line shop.

Institute of Phytobiophysics (UK)

01534 738737
www.phytobiophysics.co.uk
Mail-order and on-line ordering. Advice and postal consultation service also available.

Aromatherapy products

All the following companies have developed special ranges or products to help you sleep; all use high-quality essential oils at therapeutic concentrations. Most can be ordered on-line. Aromatherapy burners can be ordered on-line from: www.quinessence.co.uk and www.riobeauty.com. Have fun!

Aromatherapy Associates

0207 371 9878 (UK orders)
www.aromatheapyassociates.com
One of the top brands, established for 28 years. They primarily supply spas and health clinics. I use their Deep Relax bath oil; their Relax pillar candle is also one of the best. Mail world-wide; also

available from SPNK stores, Harvey Nichols and Fortnum & Mason in London.
US customers, contact:

Aromatherapy Associates

972-712-9980
e-mail: aromatherapyus@aol.com

Aroma Therapeutics™ (UK)

01458 835925
www.aroma.co.uk
Created by jet-setting international model, Anastasia Alexander. Sleep-Enhancer range for bath and body plus Sleep-Enhancer candle. Mail-order world-wide.

Comfort & Joy® (UK)

01367 850278
www.comfortandjoy.co.uk
e-mail: merrie@comfortandjoy.co.uk
Tiny family company with a passion to help, specializing in hand-made face and body care products from organic ingredients. Range includes relaxing bath oils and individually blended oils for various stress/hormonal/emotional complaints. Recommended.

Dream Line™ (UK)

www.thepuresleep.com
Snazzy range developed with the help of a sleep scientist. Cloud 9 bath soak, Water Bed bath oil; Restless Nights dry body oil; Drowsy Dew acupressure gel; Bed Socks foot oil; Wake-Up shower gel (thoroughly recommended after a hard night's not sleeping). Available in major Boots stores. For more info, see website.

Elemis (UK)

0208 954 8033 (for stockists and mail-order)
www.elemis.com
Three products for sleep: de-stress massage oil; pure lavender essential oil; and the wonderful Lavender eye pillow. Also available in over 600 spas world-wide.

Materia Aromatica

0208 392 9868 (UK orders)
www.materia-aromatica.com
e-mail: info@materia-aromatica.com
Organic and wild crafted essential oils, including Peaceful Night bath oil. Ring for catalogue. They also have blends for Indian head massage, a chakra blend for chakra healing, meridian blends to activate *chi* in a specific meridian point, and aromatherapy oil soft travel bags. Their newsletter contains nice-to-know snippets. On-line ordering. Mail world-wide.

Quinessence

01530 838358 (UK orders)
01530 814171 (help line)
www.quinessence.com
e-mail: enquiries@quinessence.com
Established for over 20 years, very respected, knowledgeable and committed brand; very good value. Restful Sleep bath oil. On-line shop. Mail world-wide.

Origins

0800 731 4039 (for UK stockists)
www.origins.com
Part of Estée Lauder Group. Sensory Therapy® range, chic and developed with the help of sleep scientists: milk bath; body lotion; pillow mist; bedside diffuser; spot gel; night cream. Widely available internationally, including in the US. Their bedtime diffuser is permanently under my pillow.

Allison England Aromatherapy (UK)

01353 699236
www.allison.england.dial.pipex.com
e-mail: allison.england@dial.pipex.com
Specialist range of aromatherapy products for pregnancy, babies and new mothers (and fathers). Lovely products, on-line ordering and gift-wrapping service.

Mind/body/spirit bookshops

Books, meditation/relaxing music/New Age CDs and cassette tapes:

The Cygnus Review (UK)

0845 456 1577
www.cygnus-books.co.uk
e-mail: info@cygnus-books.co.uk
Popular free (very useful) body/mind/spirit books review magazine; order titles reviewed at discount prices on-line or by mail-order. Over 1,200 titles stocked. Lovely website.

Esoteric Centre (UK)

0207 379 4554
www.watkinsbooks.com
e-mail: service@watkinsbooks.com
Body/mind/spirit cornucopia, where 'magic meets therapy and divination meets sacred ritual'. Therapies and courses as well as music/meditation/self-help CDs and tapes, aromatherapy oils, crystals and much more.

Watkins Bookshop (UK)

0207 836 2182
The original UK body/mind/spirit specialist bookshop. Hold around 20,000 titles in stock. Mail world-wide.

The Inner Bookshop (UK)

01865 245301

www.innerbookshop.com

e-mail: mail@innerbookshop.com

Hold around 20,000 new and second-hand titles in stock. Ring for catalogue. Music/meditation/self-help CDs and tapes. Mail worldwide.

Plus:

The ideal gift for the insomniac. *Hello Midnight, the Insomniac's Literary Bedside Companion* by Deborah Bishop and David Levy, published by Touchstone Books, available from on-line bookshops such as www.amazon.com/co.uk; or www.bookcloseouts.com. Includes words of wisdom from famous insomniacs, tongue-in-cheek suggestions for getting to sleep, amusing guides to sleep aids, etc., etc.

Meditation/music/self-help CDs and cassette tapes

Sounds True (US)

00-1-800-333-9185

www.soundstrue.com

e-mail: info@soundstrue.com (product information) or customer-service@soundstrue.com (questions re orders).

Unique audio, video and music publishing company for the inner life, encompassing everything from meditation and the humanities to relationships, and voice and sound works. Huge range of recordings from well-known mind/body/spirit artists, experts and teachers. Catalogue and on-line shop.

Meditation – a complete workout for the mind by Richard Lawrence

0207 736 4187

www.richardlawrence.co.uk

e-mail: orders@innerpotential.org

Bliss CDs (UK)

01865 340981
www.blissfulmusic.com
Joni Mitchell meets meditation. A Thousand Angels (soothing) and their latest CD; Bliss (more up-beat) are my recommendations. Their *Journey* album (purely instrumental) is very calming, and was composed to meditate by.

Symbiosis (UK)

0208 948 5880 (orders)
0208 781 0755 (24-hour music line)
www.symbiosis-music.com
e-mail: relax@symbiosis-music.com
Specialist musicians with a mission to create ultra-relaxing music that works. Touching The Cloud is popular with complementary therapists.

Soundworks (UK)

01798 812559
www.sacredsound.net
Sound therapy CDs. Slow, sonorous, vaguely Tibetan-like compositions that may sound strange if you are new to this kind of thing. Current titles are Chakra Balance (my favourite, includes drumbeat sequences), Crystal and Stone, and Dreamscape.
Plus:
Pilgrim self-help tapes – page 253
Inner Talk self-help CDs and tapes – page 253

Helpful organizations

Nutritional/complementary health clinics

Allergy UK (The British Allergy Foundation)
Helpline: 0208 303 8525 (9 a.m.–9 p.m. weekdays; 10 a.m.–1 p.m. weekends)
www.allergyuk.org
Patient information charity. Provide support, advice, fact sheets and help to find your nearest allergy clinic/specialist.

The Aesculus Clinic (UK)
01202 660044
e-mail: electrodoc2@aol
Run by Anthony Scott-Morley, one of the UK's foremost bio-energy medicine experts, who studied under original pioneer, Dr Voll. The clinic offers a range of other complementary therapies.

Body Wisdom Clinic (UK)
07939 100797
www.jenniferharper.com
Run by Dr Jennifer Harper. Multi-disciplinary approach blending an eclectic mix of Eastern and Western natural therapies.

Food and Mood Project (UK)

01273 478108 (answer machine)
www.foodandmood.org
e-mail: amanda.geary@foodandmood.org
Run by Amanda Geary. Specialist food and mood-disorder clinic.

The Hale Clinic (UK)

0870 167 6667 (appointment line)
www.haleclinic.com
100 practitioners including medical doctors, and over 40 complementary therapies available. Offer an integrated approach; treating insomnia is a particular specialism. Helpful new patient advisory service. Ring for more details, or visit their website, which includes an A-Z of therapies offered.

Integrated Medical Centre (UK)

0207 224 5111 (clinic)
0207 224 5141 (shop/order line)
www.dr-ali.co.uk
Dr Ali is a well-known integrated health expert, who combines alleopathic, complementary and Ayurvedic medicine. Ask for a 'gatekeeper session' with Dr Ali, who will then recommend treatment with his other complementary therapists if necessary. Nutritional and Ayurvedic health supplements, and Dr Ali's books are available from their shop and by mail-order.

The Nutrition Clinic (UK)

01626 364722
www.thenutritionclinic.com
e-mail: antony@thenutritionclinic.com
Run by Antony Haynes. Specialize in the use of nutritional treatments for mood, stress and neurological disorders. Offer full range of diagnostic tests, including adrenal/cortisol assays. Clinic also at 1 Harley St, London, Mondays and Tuesdays.

Wimbledon Clinic of Natural Medicine (UK)

0208 543 5477

www.wimbledonclinic.co.uk

Run by Thomas Marshall-Manifold – bio-energetic specialist, TCM practitioner, chiropracter, acupuncturist and nutritional expert. Over 25 years' experience. Excellent website.

Spring Gardens Clinic (UK)

01227 761000

www.nature-cure.co.uk

Run by Tom Greenfield, naturopath, craniosacral therapist and fellow of the Institute for Human Individuality; specialist in blood groups and their contribution to health and disorders.

Diagnostic testing, hormones, etc.

The easiest and best way to have diagnostic tests is through a complementary practitioner, who will have access to specialist laboratories and can help analyse the results and suggest an appropriate treatment protocol. If you want to go solo, or suggest some to your practitioner, the following laboratories offer a range of tests.

Great Smokies Diagnostic Laboratory (US)

www.gsdl.com

Offer the most comprehensive testing of hormones, etc. On-line global service. Many practitioners use them.

Individual Wellbeing Diagnostic Laboratories (UK)

0207 730 7010

www.iwdl.net

e-mail: info@iwdl.net

Offer comprehensive range of diagnostic tests including allergy and hormonal tests. Many practitioners use them.

Yorktest Laboratories (UK)

Freephone 0800 074 6185 (for kits)
01904 777722
www.yorktest.com
e-mail: info@yorktest.com
European leader in food-intolerance testing, using latest blood-sampling techniques. Recommended by nutritionist Patrick Holford.

Stacktheme Ltd (UK)

01259 743200
www.stacktheme.com
European agents for Dr Peter D'Adamo's 'Eat Right for Your Type' diet. Offer blood-group diagnostic kits. Also sell D'Adamo's books/blood-friendly nutritional supplements, and Solgar vitamins. See website for contact details for Europe/rest of the world.
Also: Higher Nature (page 254) offer a saliva test service for hormone analysis.
Plus:
The Nutrition Clinic (page 266) offers a full range of health/nutrition/hormonal diagnostic tests.
Wimbledon Clinic of Natural Medicine (page 267) offers a full range of health/nutritional/hormonal diagnostic tests.
Spring Gardens Clinic (page 267) offers comprehensive diagnostic testing, complete medical and well-being bio-assays, blood-group testing and analysis, and Dr Luscher's stress colour test.
See also Allergy UK, page 265.

Sleep organizations (UK)

The British Sleep Society

www.sleeping.org
e-mail: enquiries@sleeping.org.uk
Will provide general practitioners with an up-to-date list of sleep clinics.

British Snoring and Sleep Apnoea Association (BSSAA)

0800 085 1097 (general/help line)
www.britishsnoring.com
e-mail: info@britishsnoring.com
Excellent patient support group. Provide information packs, advice on where to go and what medical treatment/products may help. Informative website includes self-diagnosis on what kind of snorer you (or your partner) are.

Narcolepsy Association UK (UKAN)

0207 721 8904 (message-taking service)
www.narcolepsy.org.uk
e-mail: info@narcolepsy.org.uk
Self-help association for narcoleptics and their families dedicated to the benefit, relief and education of persons suffering from narcolepsy. Excellent website.

Sleep advisory services

NHS Direct (UK)

0845 4647
Will help you find sleep centres/clinics/sleep disorder centres near you, plus will send you insomnia leaflet and booklet *How to Cope with Sleep*.

Sleep Assessment and Advisory Service

Prof. C Idzikowski, BSc PhD CPsychol FBPsS
0845 1300 933
www.sleepspecialist.co.uk
e-mail: office@sleepspecialist.co.uk

The Jetlag Clinic

0207 584 9779
www.drdavidoconnell.co.uk
e-mail: info@drdavidoconnell.co.uk

Private clinic run by Dr David O'Connell. Specializes in individual management and treatment of jet-lag (before and after) for business-people, etc. undertaking long-haul flights. Prescribes melatonin and sells light visors. Also sells his book *Jetlag, How to Beat It* – primarily for normal sleepers but very useful.

Sleep clinics

London Sleep Centre

0207 725 0523
www.londonsleepcentre.com
e-mail: info@londonsleepcentre.com
The UK's first comprehensive private sleep centre, marrying the latest scientific research and assessment methods with the multi-faceted 'Sigma' approach to treatment, incorporating both medical and holistic therapies. Aim to return you to normal sleeping patterns.

BUPA Hospitals

The BUPA hospitals below all list 'Sleep Studies' among their services. You will need to contact them to find out whether they specifically treat insomnia. If they do not, they may be able to point you in the right direction. The link at the bottom has contact details for all their hospitals. The easiest way is to e-mail the customer service address that is shown for each hospital.
BUPA Alexandra
BUPA Bristol
BUPA Dunedin
BUPA Fylde Coast
BUPA Gatwick Park
BUPA Harpenden
BUPA Hastings
BUPA Hull & East Riding
BUPA Manchester
BUPA Methley Park

BUPA Norwich
BUPA Portsmouth
Contact Details:
http://www.bupahospitals.co.uk/asp/contactlist.asp
Head Office:
BUPA House, 15–19 Bloomsbury Way, London, WC1
www.bupa.com
For sleep/insomnia websites, see page 238.
For American and Australian sleep organizations, see page 284.

Complementary health organizations

Institute of Complimentary Medicine (UK)

0207 237 5165
www.icmedicine.co.uk
Registered charity. Hold BRCP (British Register of Complementary Practitioners). Practitioner-search on website will give you all qualified practitioners registered with them.

Holistic Medicine Resource Centre

www.holisticmed.com
Directories of practitioners: www.holisticmed.com/www/directory.html
The website you've been looking for. Global resource site for holistic medicine. Find whatever therapy you need, whoever you want, wherever you are.

Aromatherapy

International Federation of Aromatherapists

0208 742 2605
www.ifaroma.org
e-mail: office@ifaroma.org
Worldwide aromatherapy association; publish their own journal. Provide practitioner details. Website practioner-search.

The Internet Guide to Aromatherapy
www.fragrant.demon.co.uk
Global aromatherapy website. Includes lengthy lists of suppliers and practitioners arranged by country: UK, US, Australia, rest of world.

Autogenics

The British Autogenic Society

www.autogenic-therapy.co.uk
Professional and regulatory body for UK Autogenic practitioners. Website practitioner-search.

Ayurvedic medicine

Ayurvedic Medical Association UK

c/o The Hale Clinic (see page 266)
www.ayurveda.co.uk
All members are qualified Ayurvedic doctors who have received six years' training. Send SAE to the Hale Clinic for list of registered doctors; visit website for practitioner-search.

The British Biomagnetic Association

The Williams Clinic, Torquay, Devon
01803 293346
e-mail: secretary@britishbiomagneticassoc.fsnet.co.uk
Affiliated to the PIA in Japan. Only train qualified practitioners (osteopaths, acupuncturists, homoeopaths, etc.). Provide details of your nearest practitioner.

Chiropractic

General Chiropractic Council

0207 713 5155

www.gcc-uk.org

e-mail: enquiries@gcc-uk.org

UK's statutory chiropractic body with regulatory powers. Publish leaflets including register of chiropracters. Over 2,000 listed. Website practitioner-search.

Herbalism

National Institute of Medical Herbalists (UK)

01392 426022

www.nimh.org.uk

e-mail: nimh@ukexter.freeserve.co.uk

Largest organization, with over 650 members (3–5 years' training required). Phone for details of local practitioners. Limited website practitioner-search also.

Homeopathy

British Homeopathic Association

08704 443 950

www.trusthomeopathy.org

Registered charity providing information about medical homoeopathy (medical doctors and vets qualified in homoeopathy). Ring for information pack which includes list of practitioners; or use practitioner-search on website.

Society of Homeopaths

01604 621400

www.homeopathy-soh.org

Society of professional homoeopaths. Ring for practitioner list, or use practitioner-search on website.

Hypnotherapy

British Hypnotherapy Association

0207 7723 4443

www.british-hynotherapy-association.org

Well-known hypnotherapy organization. Strict membership conditions, including four years' mandatory training. Ring for information booklet and details of nearest hypnotherapists. Website has useful introduction to hypnotherapy, and full explanation of their society and members' qualifications.

British Society for Medical and Dental Hypnosis

www.bsmdh.org

e-mail: nat.office@bsmdh.org

National organization of NHS doctors, dentists and health professionals, trained in hypnosis.

National Register of Hypnotherapists and Psychotherapists

0800 161 3823 (freephone)

www.nrhp.co.uk.

Hold register for hypnotherapists and psychotherapists trained to Council of Pyschotherapists' standards. Provide details of local practitioners. Website practitioner-search.

Massage

General Council of Massage Therapists

0151 430 8199

e-mail: gcmt@btconnect.com

The Shiatsu Society UK

0845 1304560

www.shiatsu.org

e-mail: admin@shiatsu.org

Hold UK register for qualified shiatsu practitioners. Ring for information and nearest practitioner. Practitioner website search also.

Meditation/spiritual healing/retreats

The Atherius Society

0207 736 4187
All-embracing metaphysical and spiritual healing society.
Publications, CDs, workshops and absent healing.

The Inner Potential Centre

0207 731 1067
www.innerpotential.org
e-mail: bookings@innerpotential.org
Part of Atherius Society. Centre for personal development. Courses
include meditation, yoga, sound and colour therapy.

National Federation of Spiritual Healers

01932 783164
www.nfsh.org.uk
Established healing organization. Conduct healing and provide
details of practitioners registered with them. Clear website and
practitioner-search.

Global Retreat Centre

01865 343 551
www.globalretreatcentre.org.uk
e-mail: info@globalretreatcentre.com
International residential/retreat centre for Brahma Kumaris World
Spiritual University. Splendid setting and facilities. Hold regular
events and meditation courses. No fees; donations welcome.

The Brahma Kumaris also have retreat centres in Australia, Italy,
Rajasthan and New York. See www.bkwsu.com.

London Buddhist Centre

0845 458 4716

www.lbc.org.uk and www.londonbuddhistcentre.com

e-mail: info@lbc.org.uk and info@londonbuddhistcentre.com

Part of the Friends of the Western Buddhist Order (FWBO). Teach meditation, hold introductory meditation evenings and lunchtime classes, and organize meditation weekends and retreats.

The Retreat Company

0116 259 9211

www.theretreatcompany.com

e-mail: timeout@retreat.co.uk

Provide information service on worldwide retreats, well-being/holistic courses, etc; teach meditation; offer Ayurvedic treatments. *See also* The Practice, page 280.

Transcendental Meditation

08705 143733

www.t-m.org.uk

e-mail: info@t-m.org.uk

UK headquarters. Give details of nearest centre. Comprehensive website includes links to TM centres worldwide.

TM – US

www.tm.org

TM – Australia

www.tmprogram.com.au

See also Sounds True, page 263.

Nutrition

British Association of Nutritional Therapy

0870 606 1284

www.bant.org.uk

Website practitioner search

Institute of Optimum Nutrition

0208 877 9993

www.ion.co.uk

Founded by nutritionist Patrick Holford. Their nutritionists offer very thorough nutritional/holistic check-ups. Ring for info and directory of qualified consultants, or use practitioner-search on website.

Psychotherapy

Centre for Transpersonal Psychology

0207 724 9842

www.transpersonalcentre.co.uk

e-mail: enquiries@transpersonalcentre.co.uk

Transpersonal Psychology offers a spiritual approach to psychotherapy. A gentle method of self-analysis, which acknowledges there is something beyond the personality. Helpful for complicated insomniacs like myself, and embraces, among other elements, dreams and feelings, the work of C G Jung, and Buddist philosophy. Website contains details of workshops and practitioner-search.

Tai Chi

Tai Chi Union for Great Britain

www.taichiunion.com

Official Tai Chi union; over 400 registered qualified practitioners. Excellent website with practitioner-search; comprehensive link section.

See also Tai Chi UK, page 282.

Traditional Chinese Medicine

British Acupuncture Council

0208 735 0400

www.acupuncture.org.uk

e-mail: info@acupuncture.org.uk

UK's main regulatory body for TCM acupuncturists; over 2,200 qualified practitioners registered. Website practitioner-search.

Register of Chinese Herbal Medicine

01603 623994

www.rchm.co.uk

e-mail: herbmed@rchm.co.uk

Register for qualified herbal TCM practitioners. Supply local lists. Website practitioner search.

Yoga

British Wheel of Yoga

01529 306851

www.bwy.org.uk

Governing body for Yoga (Hatha) in the UK. Ring or visit website for county representative, who will put you in touch with local yoga teachers.

Viniyoga Britain

0870 1302785

www.viniyoga.co.uk or www.yogastudies.org

Websites include list of UK practitioners.

Experts and practitioners

UK

My personal list of complementary health experts and practitioners I have consulted or have received treatment from.

Aromatherapy/Massage

Marie-Louise Carey-Morgan

01491 680 365

Clare Maxwell-Hudson Massage Therapy Institute

0208 208 1637
www.cmhmassage.co.uk

Stewart Mitchell

01647 433842
e-mail: instituteofch@aol.com
Naturopathic and anthroposophical practice; massage expert.

Autogenics

Christine Pinch

01646 694149
e-mail: chris@pinch.demon.co.uk
Has a particular interest in sleep problems and insomnia.

z z z z

Jenny Cuff
0118 986 6987
e-mail: jennycuff@aol.com

Ayurveda

Sebastian Pole Lic OHM, Ayur HC, MRCHM, MURHP
01225 466944
www.blueskyclinic.co.uk
Ayurvedic and Chinese medical practitioner.

The Practice
0116 259 9211
www.thetreatcompany.com/thepractice
e-mail: info@thetreatcompany.com
Residential 2- to 5-day breaks (held at Tor Retreat, Canterbury); personalized specialized detox and other Ayurvedic treatments, including *Shirodhara*. Ayurvedic meals, meditation classes, yoga/tai chi also.

Bio-energy medicine

Thomas Marshall-Manifold DC., Lic.Ac., Lic.O.H.M., D.Sc.
Wimbledon Clinic of Natural Medicine – see page 267

Anthony Scott-Morley BA; BAc.
The Aesculus Clinic – see page 265

Biomagnetic therapy

Graham Gardener
The Williams Clinic – see page 272

Chiropractic

Dr Jerome Poupel DC
01491 579204
www.thehouseofgoodhealth.co.uk

Homoeopathy

Nicky Pool, RSHom; SRN; ATPsych.

01494 485952
www.purtonhouse.com
e-mail: enquiries@purtonhouse.com

Hypnotherapy

Valerie Austin

0207 702 4900

Dr Alastair Dobbin

0131 476 6441
www.hypnodoc.co.uk
Practising GP and hypnotherapist.

Naturopathy

Tom Greenfield ND; DO; MRN; RCST

Spring Gardens Clinic – see page 267

Nutrition/food mood specialists

Antony Haynes BA (Hons); Dip ION

The Nutrition Clinic – see page 266

Amanda Geary

Food & Mood project – see page 266

Oligotherapy

Colleen O'Flaharty

0118 972 1236
www.oligotherapy.co.uk
e-mail: colleen@oligotherapy.co.uk

Personal skills
Hilary Luxton
01491 825288
Interpersonal skills specialist and Human Givens therapist.

Sound therapy
Lyz Cooper
Soundworks – see page 264

Clive Williamson
Symbiosis – see page 264

Tai Chi
Angus Clark
School of Living Movement
01647 231477
www.livingmovement.com

Michael Jacques
Tai Chi UK
0207 407 4775
www.taichiuk.co.uk

Traditional Chinese Medicine
Dr Jennifer Harper PhD; ND; MSc
See page 265

Sigyta Hart MCAA(Hong Kong). MBAcC MRCHM Kanpo
01491 873972 (appointments)
Acupuncturist and TCM doctor.

Prof Jing Hua Chen, MD

01865 766319

Consultant doctor and doctor of Traditional Chinese Medicine; specializes in the treatment of insomnia using acupuncture and Chinese Medicine. Also operates Friday surgery at the Hale Clinic in London, tel: 01923 725 1719 for bookings.

Also: Thomas Marshall-Manifold and Anthony Scott-Morley (see pages 267 and 265)

Transpersonal psychology

Judith O'Hagan

0208 995 2250 (London); 01823 272227 (Taunton)

Hazel Marshall

0116 236 4256
Runs a variety of workshops.

Maggie Peters

Transformative Dreamwork Ltd
01453 872709
e-mail: maggie@maggiepeters.demon.co.uk
Dream specialist.

Viniyoga

Jane Slemeck

01491 613958
e-mail: jane@jsalearning.freeserve

American and
Australian Addresses

US

Telephone numbers, where given, are for American/Australian readers only.

American Academy of Sleep Medicine (AASM)

507-287-6006
www.aasmnet.org
America's foremost professional membership organization, dedicated to the advancement of sleep and related research. Includes countrywide search for local AASM-accredited centres and laboratories. Provide list of accredited sleep-disorder Clinics, and publish the journal *Sleep*.

The National Sleep Foundation

202-347-3471
www.sleepfoundation.org
America's best-known sleep organization, committed to improving public health by raising awareness of sleep and sleep disorders. Also supply details of sleep-disorder clinics.

American Insomnia Association (AIA)

708-492-0930
www.americaninsomniaassociation.org
e-mail: cpulvino@aasmnet.org

Patient-based organization providing information and resources to people suffering insomnia, and encourages formation of local support groups.

Dr Julia Ross Mood Cure Nutrition Clinic

415-383-3611, ext 1
www.moodcure.com

Australia

Australasian Sleep Association (ASA)

0500 500 701
www.sleepaus.on.net
e-mail: sleepaus@ozemail.com.au
Australia and New Zealand's prime scientific professional association.

Narcolepsy and Overwhelming Daytime Sleep Society of Australia (NODSS)

www.nodss.org.au
e-mail: info@nodss.org.au
National association providing support for people and their families suffering from narcolepsy and other sleep disorders. Offer 24-hour counselling and information service. See website for details.

Sleep Disorders Centre

02 9515 8630
e-mail: rrg@blackburn.med.su.oz.au

Newcastle Sleep Disorders Centre

02 4923 6833
www.newcastle.ed.aus/centre/nsdc
Excellent website with useful information on sleep disorders and insomnia.
Plus:
www.healthinsite.gov.au
www.betterhealth.vic.gov.au

Two excellent government-run health information websites. Key in 'insomnia' and you'll find lots of useful references, information and advice.

Australian Complementary Health Association

03 9650 5327
www.diversity.org.au
e-mail: diversity@diversity.org.au
Independent association of health consumers and practitioners. Excellent subscription magazine, *Diversity*, published quarterly, with practitioner search for all kinds of therapists.

Australian Acupuncture and Chinese Medicine Association Ltd

07 3846 5866; 1300 725 334 (practitioner referral services)
www.acupuncture.org.au
e-mail: aacma@acupuncture.org.au
National professional and regulatory association for acupuncture and Traditional Chinese Medicine; represents over 80 per cent of qualified practitioners. Website practitioner search.

National Herbalists Association of Australia

02 9555 8885
www.nhaa.org.au
e-mail: nhaa@nhaa.org.au
Leading professional association of medical herbalists, established in the 1920s. Website practitioner search (click on 'referrals') or by telephone. Wonderful links section for medical herb buffs, or anyone interested in herbal medicine.

Sounds Wonderful Pty Ltd

03 9844 3933
www.chrisjames.net or www.sacredsound.com
e-mail: admin@chrisjames.net
International sound therapist; everyone should experience him once.

Your sleep diary

The sleep diary here should only take a minute or so to do. It's designed to elucidate your 'sleep architecture' – the term used for how you physically sleep – and to provide an indication of how your sleep affects your mood and performance, and how you are generally faring. To show you how it works, it has been filled in for real by an insomniac friend. A few points:

1. The diary is deliberately generalized; *don't* look at the clock during the night, or feel you have to be too precise. It's not a test or statistically relevant.
2. Complete Part A of the diary for each previous night as soon as you wake up, or as early the next day as possible – your last night's sleep may be vividly imprinted on your memory when you get out of bed, but has a habit of becoming a hazy memory as the day wears on. Complete Part B ideally in the evening, or when you remember.
3. The diary is primarily for *you*. If you see a sleep doctor/clinic, they will want you to fill their own in, which may be more specific.
4. Medications include drugs, herbal remedies, supplements, etc. taken specifically to help you sleep. If you are using a sleep aid, record that. Including them in your sleep diary helps you to see how they are working.
5. If you want to calculate your sleep efficiency (page 200), divide the time spent asleep by time spent in bed, and multiply by 100.

z z z z

6. Be as honest with yourself as you can. You can actually have a bad night and feel OK; so don't over-egg the downside, and try not to underestimate how much you've slept. It's bad enough anyway.
7. If you are a first-time sleep-diary person, it's a very good idea also to track what you eat and drink; one nutritionist told me how he managed to cure someone's insomnia by getting them to stop drinking strong tea. More work, but could be worth it.
8. The Comments column is for extenuating circumstances or anything that might be relevant to the previous night's sleep – from barking dogs and worries at work to how hot you were and midnight binges.

Part A

Night	*Fri*
Date	*19th Sept 2003*
Medications taken	*none*
What time did you get into bed?	*11p.m.*
Lights off?	*11.30 p.m.*
About how long did it take to fall asleep?	*20 mins*
About how many times did you wake up?	*4*
About how long were you awake each time?	*10 mins, 1 hour,* *10 mins, 5 mins*
Your final wake-up time?	*6 a.m.*
When did you get up?	*7 a.m.*
Total time spent in bed?	*8*
Total hours of sleep?	*4.45*
Sleep efficiency?	*4.45/8 x 100 55%*
Sleep rating: How was your sleep? (0 = dreadful, 5 = excellent):	*3*

Comments:
I felt very antsy, hot and restless so I knew on getting into bed that I wouldn't have a good night's sleep. Feels like a hormonal thing. Got up twice during night.

Part B

How did you feel the next day?

0	5	
extremely tired	rested	*4*
lethargic	energized	*3*
dull-witted/confused	mentally sharp	*3*
depressed	cheerful	*3*
anxious	confident	*2*
frustrated	relaxed	*2*

What kind of day did you have?

0	5	
awful	great	*3*

z z z z

Bibliography

Sleep and insomnia

Beating Insomnia (includes CD with guided progressive relaxation exercise), Prof Chris Idzikowski (Newleaf Publishers)

Learn to Sleep Well Kit (includes CD), Prof Chris Idzikowski (Duncan Baird)

– These books by Professor Idzikowski are the two best general books on sleep/insomnia

Counting Sheep, Paul Martin (HarperCollins)

Doctor, I Can't Sleep, Dr Adrian Williams (Amberwood Publishing Ltd)

Getting a Good Night's Sleep, Fiona Johnston (Sheldon Press)

Help Your Baby to Sleep (National Childbirth Trust), Penny Hames, Thorsons

Insomnia, Your Questions Answered, Dr Dilys Davies (Vega)

Jetlag, How to Beat It, Dr David O'Connell (Ascendant Publishing)

Learn to Sleep Well, Sheila Lavery (Gaia Books Ltd) – also recommended

The Promise of Sleep, William C Dement with Christopher Vaughan (Pan Books)

Say Goodnight to Insomnia, Gregg D Jacobs, PhD, (Owl Books) – highly recommended

Seven Days to a Perfect Night's Sleep, Debra L Gordon (Griffin Original)

z z z z

Nutrition

The Mood Cure, Dr Julia Ross (Thorsons)
Optimum Nutrition for the Mind, Patrick Holford (Piatkus)
– Both fascinating and essential reading
Eat Right 4 Your Type, Dr Peter D'Adamo (Penguin Putnam Inc)
The Food and Mood Handbook, Amanda Geary (Thorsons)
The New Shopper's Guide to Organic Food, Lynda Brown (Fourth Estate)
The Optimum Nutrition Bible, Patrick Holford (Piatkus)

Complementary medicine

Liberation, Barefoot Doctor (Element)
Vibrational Medicine for the 21st Century, Richard Gerber MD (Piatkus)
– Two great books
Aromatherapy and Massage for Mother and Baby, Allison England (Vermillion)
Autogenic Therapy, Self-help for Mind and Body, Jane Bird and Christine Pinch (Newleaf)
Bach Flower Therapy, Mechthild Scheffer (Thorsons)
Bach Flower Remedies, A Step-by-Step Guide (Element)
The Book of Ayurveda, a Guide to Personal Wellbeing, Judith H Morrison (Gaia Books Ltd)
The Complete Book of Massage, Clare Maxwell-Hudson (Dorling Kindersley)
The Complete Illustrated Guide to Massage, Stewart Mitchell (Element)
Curing Insomnia Naturally with Chinese Medicine, Bob Flaw (Blue Poppy Press Inc.)
The 5-minute Meditator, by Eric Harrison (Piatkus)
The Illustrated Encyclopedia of Feng Shui, Lillian Too (Element)
The Illustrated Guide of Tai Chi, Angus Clark (Element)
The Meditation Plan, Richard Lawrence (Piatkus)
Nine Ways to Body Wisdom, Dr Jennifer Harper (Thorsons)
Secrets of Yoga, Jennie Bittleston (Dorling Kindersley)

Self-Hypnosis, Valerie Austin (Thorsons)

Simply Ayurveda, Bharti Vyas with Jane Warren (Thorsons)

The Sivananda Book of Meditation, The Sivananda Yoga Vedanta Centre (Gaia Books Ltd)

What Really Works, Susan Clark (Thorsons) – Excellent general 'insider's guide to natural health'

Psychotherapy

Dreamwork – Using your dreams as the way to self-discovery and personal development, Maggie Peters (Gaia Books Ltd)

Journey in Depth, Barbara Somers with Ian Gordon-Brown (Archive Publishing)

The Joy of Burnout, Dr Dina Glouberman (Hodder Mobius)

Acknowledgements

This book has brought me in contact with many sincerely good people, whose help, stories, advice and co-operation have enriched me personally in many different ways, and who have collectively made writing this book a privilege. I thank them all most fondly.

First and foremost, to my fellow insomniacs – the people who have made this book come alive – for sharing their stories with me; my heartfelt gratitude and best wishes to all. My heartfelt gratitude and appreciative thanks, also, to the various experts I have consulted along the way, who have each contributed so selflessly.

For their various contributions I should like to especially thank: Valerie Austin, Sue Beecher, Jenny Bullough, Marie-Louise Carey-Morgan, Dr Alastair Dobbin, Dr Irshaad Ebrahim, Graham Gardener, Dr Diane Glauberman, Tom Greenfield, Dr Jennifer Harper, Grant Healey, Prof. Jim Horne, Simone de Lacy, Daphne Lambert, Richard Lawrence, Stephanie Leonard, Geoff Lyth, Clare Maxwell-Hudson, Sherry Moran, Anthony Mossop, Maggie Peters, Christopher Perry, Jane Slemeck, Tony Pinkus, Dr Jerome Poupel, Gare Ridgeway, Anthony Rodale, Anthony Scott-Morley, Sarah Sewell, Sarah Stacey, Simon Wright, Eldon Taylor, Dr Adrian Williams and Charles Wells.

I should also like to pay a special tribute to: Carol, for her diligent work surfing the web; Prof. Chris Idzikowski for his generosity and expert advice; Nick and Michael, for their much needed help, support and feedback; James Self for his kindness; Jackie and Steve for making me feel at home during my stay at Kilvert's Cottage in Winforton; likewise to Tina and Jessica and their lovely cottage in Turville. A very special thank you, too, to my agent, Rosemary Scoular, for her guidance, but most of all for believing I could do it.

I should, in addition, like to thank Newleaf publishers for allowing me to reprint the illustration on page 5 from *Beating Insomnia*; and Piatkus publishers for allowing me to reprint short extracts on pages 117 and 136 from Patrick Holford's *Optimum Nutrition Bible* and *Optimum Nutrition for the Mind*.

On a personal level, I have never had to rely on people so much in my life. For Joanna and Catey, for always being there for me, my best love to both (and for baby Buzz, too). For my brother Barry, for his unstinting support and good care throughout, my love and sincere thanks. For Christiane, my heartfelt love. For Judith, for staying the course, and for Nicky, who brightened up my life more than she knew, my sincere appreciation and warmest thanks. Last but by no means least, for my editor, Wanda Whiteley, for her sweet nature and for understanding and supporting me throughout, affectionate gratitude and life-long thanks.

Sharing your life with a writer is no easy task; sharing your life with someone who has insomnia and who is also writing a book, is beyond the pale. For Rick, the unsung hero of this book, the person who had to bear the brunt and suffer alongside me every long step of the way, for his patience and understanding, my eternal gratitude and love. I am getting better, promise.

Index

z z z z

z z z z

z z z z

z z z z

z z z z

z z z z